D1606070

Whips & Kisses

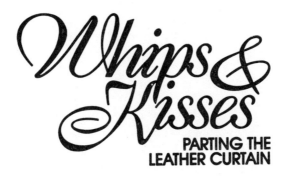

Whips & Kisses

PARTING THE LEATHER CURTAIN

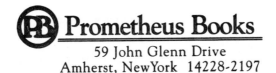

Mistress Jacqueline

**AS TOLD TO CATHERINE TAVEL
AND ROBERT H. RIMMER**

Prometheus Books

59 John Glenn Drive
Amherst, New York 14228-2197

With a few exceptions, the names of the characters in this book have been changed.

95 94   5

Library of Congress Cataloging-in-Publication Data

Mistress Jacqueline, 1951-
   Whips and kisses : parting the leather curtain / by Mistress Jacqueline as told to Catherine Tavel and Robert H. Rimmer.

      p.   cm.
   ISBN 0-87975-656-X
   1. Mistress Jacqueline, 1951-   . 2. Sadomasochism—United States—Biography.
I. Tavel, Catherine. II. Rimmer, Robert H., 1917-   . III. Title.
HQ79.M57   1991
306.77'5—dc20   90-27046
                                                                             CIP

Printed in the United States of America on acid-free paper.

To the boys at the Queen Mary, circa 1981–1985
(you know who you are)

The relation of love to pain is one of the most difficult problems, and yet one of the most fundamental in the whole range of sexual psychology. Why is it that love inflicts, and even seeks to inflict, pain? Why is it that love suffers pain, and even seeks to suffer it?

Havelock Ellis
Love and Pain

Contents

Foreword

Sadism and masochism are forms of sexual behavior that are not very well understood. The professional literature is notably lacking in description and analysis of them. This is unfortunate because there is a large sadomasochistic culture that only rarely comes to public attention. The two phenomena are closely related since their practitioners tend to satisfy each other's needs. Since at least two people are involved in an S&M relationship (as it is properly known), it exists in the context of a social organization—there is an organized subculture in our society concerned with S&M and composed of people who either like to punish others or enjoy being punished. Usually such social organizations also engage in fantasies, which often are so carefully planned that they resemble theatrical productions.

This book is an autobiography of a dominatrix, and the dominatrix is an important aspect of many S&M relationships. Many men want to be dominated by a woman, even punished by a woman. Many of the men in society who have this masochistic desire spend much of their time dominating others and the S&M world has many a business executive and white-collar professional in their groups. Often masochists are dominant in other settings and using S&M to express a different side of their personality.

What kind of a woman becomes a dominatrix? What are her feelings? How did she enter the field? Who are her clients? How do her clients respond? What does she tell her friends? These are the questions Mistress Jacqueline attempts to answer for us.

We know so little about what goes into making up the sexual orientation of each of us that the more we can explore various aspects of the sexual scene the better our understanding of it will be. In telling us about her clients, Mistress Jacqueline emphasizes the great enigma of human sexuality. In telling us about herself we can better understand the complex motives and drives that lead someone into becoming a dominatrix. This book marks the fourth in a series dealing with "sexual occupations," the purpose of which is to give us insights into the variety of sexual behavior. We all can learn a lot from reading what Mistress Jacqueline has to say about ourselves as humans and about the human condition in general.

Vern L. Bullough

Introduction

Until a few years ago, I didn't know very much about S&M. If the truth be told, I wasn't even sure how to pronounce "dominatrix" correctly. And what *was* S&M anyway? In my mind, it was pain and perversion, sick and deviant. Boy, was I wrong.

One day in March 1989 I came home to find a letter neatly typed on bright pink stationery. It was from a lady named "Mistress Jacqueline." As women working in the vast universe of erotica, we were both members of a support group called "The Pink Ladies Social Club." Jacqueline was responding to an announcement in a recent newsletter that Robert Rimmer and I were recruiting adult-film actresses to give brief biographies for a book we were hoping to compile in the wake of our work on Jerry Butler's autobiography, *Raw Talent*. Jacqueline was interested in being part of that project, but she also wanted to discuss our collaborating on her own life story.

I had decidedly mixed feelings on this proposal. Jaundiced by preconceived notions and sexual prejudices, I had already decided that professional dominants were mean, nasty, cruel, and, oh yes, weird, too. What was the sense in even meeting her? But being a polite little authoress, I gave Jacqueline a call. To my surprise, she sounded as pleasant and courteous as she did in her note. Not only wasn't she horrid, she was obviously very intelligent. Jacqueline was a former fifth-grade schoolteacher turned clinical psychologist turned dominatrix. She held a master's degree in psychology, and was also planning on getting her Ph.D. soon. I still wasn't sold on the idea of doing her book, but I saw no harm in at least seeing Jacqueline the next time she came to her native New York City from Los Angeles, where she now resided.

Jacqueline was nothing like I'd expected. She wasn't dripping in leather, but dressed in a comfortable, peach-shaded sweatsuit and sneakers. A tiny woman with piles of blonde hair that cascaded over her shoulders, she wore very little makeup and looked almost childlike. Perhaps it was her inquisitive sea-green eyes, but I felt comfortable with Jacqueline almost immediately.

In the bright vinyl coffeeshop of the Edison Hotel we sat, strangers in one way, but bonded by our allegiance to the Pink Ladies. We discussed the repercussions of being women in a field that the rest of the world considers a bit bizarre. Although neither of us had done hardcore sex in adult films, Jacqueline had made some B&D (bondage and domination) efforts. The very nature of being a professional dominatrix and a writer, respectively, in "pornography" instantly separated us from your average, everyday career woman.

Jacqueline and I lamented the fact that we couldn't share what we *really* did for a living with certain friends and family members. The world being what it was, I couldn't tell my grandmother about my appearance on a local TV show as an "erotic scribe." She just wouldn't understand. By the same token, a "born again" former best friend couldn't appreciate any of my columns, interviews, or video reviews in the adult genre. She couldn't accept me for the person I was, either.

Jacqueline had similar experiences. No one in her family, not her parents, not even her sister, knew how she earned her pennies at that time. It's a sad brand of isolation that most people can't relate to. Never before had I met someone who shared the same fears—that family members and friends might be afraid to leave me alone with children I loved and would never dream of hurting. My "born again" buddy hinted at this, and it broke my heart. Finally, I'd met another woman who knew exactly how I felt.

Very soon after that first meeting we began working on Jacqueline's biography. It was a setup similar to the process perfected when Bob Rimmer and I pieced together *Raw Talent* with adult-film actor Jerry Butler. Jacqueline talked her story onto cassette tapes from Los Angeles and mailed them to me in Brooklyn. I, in turn, transcribed them and whisked the typed pages off to Bob Rimmer. Perhaps spoiled by Jerry's stream-of consciousness patter, Bob was extremely unhappy with the results of Jacqueline's first few tapes. I tried to convince him that Jacqueline merely expressed herself in a different way. I was certain we could get a fascinating story out of her, but some of the more intimate details of her life (such as her turbulent youth and the breakup of her marriage) were probably tough for her to unearth. We just had to remain patient. I was confident that I could infuse Jacqueline's real emotions into prose that might read rather nonchalantly and sure I could fill in the blanks with fragments from our personal conversations.

In spite of my reassurances, Bob had me send a cassette tape to Jacqueline in which he strongly voiced his discontent. I tried to soften the blow with an accompanying note, but it did no good. Jacqueline phoned me, crying hysterically. She was terribly wounded. Had her painful life story amounted to a pile of scrap? Was Bob ready to abandon the entire project? This was the ultimate form of rejection and she was deeply hurt.

Jacqueline and I called Bob separately. He was still interested in collaborating with us, but felt it would take an inordinate mountain of work to get the manuscript into shape. We were all willing to take the challenge of telling a story that would undoubtedly change a vast number of lives. After the next few tapes, Bob started calling *me* "Jacqueline" because he felt I was that much a part of her.

The tape-transcribing process is a long and frustrating one. Often, I would hear Jacqueline struggling over a difficult memory. I would want to comfort her, but it was three weeks later and the tears were long gone. She had to lose Daniel over and over again. She had to recall cruelty from a hurtful mother and an ambivalent father and survive it once more. But she did. Somehow, she did.

It didn't take long for a special friendship to blossom between this sweet dominant and myself. I was constantly in awe of her patience with my ignorance in the S&M arena. Even in videos, Jacqueline's unique brand of strong gentleness carried through. *Dresden Mistress #2* contained a scene in which she demonstrated the proper way to apply nipple clamps. "Be very careful," she warned her student, with the utmost concern in her voice. Once, while we were editing the manuscript together and reading it aloud to each other, she even showed me a virtually painless method, using herself as a guinea pig.

During our first meeting, I recall Jacqueline telling me, "I never thought I'd be doing this. I really believed I'd take my spanking fantasies with me to the grave." Few understand the sense of dread shared by those who harbor secret desires most of the world considers bizarre. I soon became intrigued with S&M. This fascination ultimately led to my feature in *Hustler* in which Jacqueline was instrumental. Not only was she the star goddess, but she also "commanded" slaves and clients to phone me with their insights to help with my research. They were more than glad to share personal B&D philosophies with others. In fact, I was amazed by the S&M community's willingness to tell their tales, but then realized that it was a relief of some sort because in our close-minded little society, there is no outlet for their fantasies. A man with a foot fetish, a woman with a fondness for rubber, are regarded as sexual freaks. Yet, these "freaks" were as polite and open and helpful —even more so—than anyone you'd meet in the street. My interviews, curiosity, and concern offered them freedom, acceptance, and the opportunity to be understood.

The sadness and joy of this almost paralyzed me. I was glad there were S&M clubs like "The Vault" where men could express their transvestite tendencies and women could be worshipped à la harmless foot massages, but felt sorry that it had to exist in a clandestine, subterranean basement. Why couldn't we be more honest about the hidden fragments of ourselves?

There's no doubt in my mind that the planet would be in much better shape if some areas of sexuality weren't such "dirty little secrets," but S&M still falls into that dubious category. Look around you. S&M is everywhere, from perfume ads to fairy tales to Ann Landers and even "I Love Lucy." Not only was TV's favorite redhead handcuffed in one episode, but she was spanked in quite a few segments and wasn't above tying up and gagging a troublesome showgirl just so she could get a part in one of Ricky's shows.

In its purest form, S&M is a game of choice played between consenting adults. Consent. That is the key word, for nothing transpires if the "slave" isn't willing to submit to a "master." S&M is selective. It is not a teenager being browbeaten by an abusive parent with a metal pipe. It is not a husband emotionally lashing a helpless spouse with an acidic tongue. In S&M frontiers, it is a grown person volunteering (and sometimes even paying generous sums of money if he or she chooses to go to a professional) for whatever personal reason. Some submissives see domination as a demonstration of love and devotion. Others, perhaps, are working out painful episodes from their childhoods and are trying to come to terms with them. After all, there is a great difference between a parental swat on the fanny and being a battered child. Another key word is *willingly*. Submissives never truly surrender their wills, nor do they give up their freedom of choice. Just the opposite. They celebrate this by participating in the scenarios of their choice.

If I hadn't worked withh Jacqueline on this book, I never would have learned all of this. I might have been like those awful "Women Against Pornography," disapproving of something I had never even witnessed. But through Jacqueline, I visited clubs, attended a meeting of the Eulenspiegel Society (an S&M association in Manhattan) and even explored the intricacies of S&M in the privacy of my own bedroom with my husband Al. There, we discovered many new things about each other. We saw each other in a new light. Although we might never indulge again, I will never forget the gentleness and mastery I found at my mate's hands, or the deep trust and love I felt. I might never have known that if we hadn't "played."

Another thing I discovered. Jacqueline and I are very much alike. Although we took separate roads in our lives, we somehow ended up in the same place. Jacqueline's strength and her need to share even the ugliest fragments of her past amazed me. I try to accomplish the same honesty in my own writing. When it came down to the fundamentals, Jacqueline and I weren't much different than most other women, except that we accepted even the oddest shreds of our sexuality and embraced them, simply because they were. The fact that they were a part of us made them valid.

To me, *Whips & Kisses* is about learning to learn, and not condemning others simply because they're different than we are.

Catherine Tavel

1

Dungeon

I am a Dominatrix. Some people call me "Goddess." And at this moment, I feel very beautiful and powerful standing in the middle of my dungeon. My studded black leather corset is cut high on my legs so that most of my taut buttocks are exposed. Leather boots cradle my thighs and fingerless gloves cover most of my arms. My long, blonde hair is teased wildly above my head, making me appear much taller than I am. Actually, I'm barely five feet, yet I tower over slave Doug, who is crouched in front of me. We are playing a game.

"Doug," I say, "How would you like to turn some of your fantasies into reality?"

"Please . . ." he almost begs.

But first, there are some things I must teach him about the sensual journey we are about to take. "To me, sadomasochism or bondage and discipline is a lifestyle. You know that I am a Dominant female. And you are obviously a submissive male." Doug nods in agreement. "I find the art of S&M erotic and stimulating. There's more to sex than just getting it on, you know. I love to tease. I love to make a man want me. Don't you want me, Doug?"

"Yes," he sighs, gazing up at me as though I am a dream. I hold my hand against Doug's full lips. Immediately, he understands and begins to lick my fingertips.

I smile. "This is about lust. But it's also about trust. Do you trust me?"

"Yes," Doug says again.

"I'm going to play with you and stimulate you, but it's important that you know I'm not going to hurt you . . .well, not too much."

Doug is naked except for a tight, black g-string. His body is slender, yet muscular. Very pleasing to the eye. "Spread your legs," I tell him. And he does. He cannot help but let tiny moans seep out when I fondle his chest, his thighs, and then his penis through the sheer material. "Powerplays. Sensuality." I coo in a melodic voice. "That's what it's all about. But I never play with anyone who doesn't want to play with me. So, Doug, would you like to play?"

"Yes."

"Are you willing to submit to me?"

"Yes."

"Then get down on your knees," I say sternly. "Now."

The room is sparsely furnished with a black lacquer cabinet, upon which sits a candelabra. Various paddles and whips decorate my walls. In one corner is a rack—very much like a high, wide corral entrance—from which I like to suspend my slaves. There is also a table, for horizontal sessions.

Doug kneels before me quite obediently as I fasten leg irons around each ankle. His hands are already chained behind his back. Sometimes I am harsh, but I never fail to compliment my slaves for their achievements. "You keep yourself in fine shape," I tell Doug. "Yes, you have a fine body, but there's one thing missing." From one of the cabinet drawers, I take out a studded collar, very much like a dog's collar. Fastening it around Doug's neck, I explain its significance. "When I put this on, it means that I own you." Doug is still on his knees. A hint of an erection is beginning to swell in his sinfully tight briefs.

"I certainly like the way you look," I say.

"Thanks, ma'am," Doug beams at me.

Although I am glad he's appreciative, Doug has overstepped his bounds as slave. "From now on," I inform him grimly, "you address me as 'Mistress.' "

"Yes, Mistress."

"Very good. But I see that you are breaking the first of my rules, which is speak when spoken to." Doug stares at me silently. "You are also breaking my second rule—no eye contact. We're not in a singles bar, you know." Doug averts his dark, serious eyes. "That's right," I continue. "Keep your eyes lowered at all times. Never look your Goddess in the eye!"

"Yes, Mistress."

I rub my body against Doug's kneeling form. The tops of my breasts spill over the leather bodice quite temptingly, eye level with his mouth. "You want to kiss these breasts," I suggest seductively.

"Yes, Mistress."

I laugh somewhat wickedly. "But you cannot kiss me, lick me, or otherwise go near me unless you have permission, slave."

Slave Doug's thick, wiry hair feels good against my fingers. With my other hand, I tickle his groin with a riding crop, continuing to state the rules of my house. "I want all parts of you attentive at all times." His cock is hardening at my crop's urging. "We've spoken before about consensuality and the mutuality of B&D. Therefore, slave, I give you a word to use, because sometimes I tend to get a bit carried away. You say, 'Mercy, Mistress.' 'Mercy, Mistress,' and I stop. Because if you scream, if you cry, if you moan or groan, I might just think you're having fun. And there's nothing that gets me hotter than your screams, slave. Understood?"

"Yes, Mistress."

"Any questions?"

"No, Mistress."

"You certainly have potential, slave." I move the creamy leather of my crop up to Doug's chest, stroking it to the accompaniment of his pleasureful sighs. "Do you like the way my crop feels?"

"Yes, Mistress."

"It has a nice caress, but it also has a nice sting. Have you ever been whipped, slave?"

"No, Mistress."

"Have you ever thought about it?"

"Yes, Mistress."

I touch Doug's face and hold it up toward me, but his eyes remain lowered. "Very good. Sometimes my slaves are reluctant to feel the kiss of my whip, but do you know what, slave? Soon they beg me for it. Anything for my touch, for my affection."

Stirring my slave to an even higher plateau of arousal, I fondle his crotch with my boot. "Do you like the way I look?"

"Yes, Mistress," he gasps in approval.

"Do you like this pretty leather I put on for you?" When Doug nods, I press my body hard into his naked skin. I know he relishes the sensation of the cool metal spikes against him. "Do you know the best part about this outfit?" I ask rhetorically. "It has a bite!"

I move to a regal, high-backed wicker chair and sit with my thighs far apart. "Next, slave, I want you to greet me in the proper manner. Do you know what that is?"

"No, Mistress."

"Move closer first. I want to rest myself on you."

Doug crawls toward me, chains jangling in a quiet music. He bends down before me. I hook one leg over his back and dig a spiked heel into his flesh. "Slave Doug, you're a very lucky slave. You have the opportunity to do what you've dreamed about for a very long time. I want you to very slowly, very loving, very sensuously worship this boot." I run my hand gracefully along the length for emphasis. "Suck it, kiss it, lick it, all the way from the bottom to the top. Do you think you can do that for me?"

"Yes, Mistress."

"If I'm not satisfied, remember that I have a whip in my hand." I crack the whip just to show my slave that I know how to use it. "Listen to it. Doesn't it have a nice sound?"

"Yes, Mistress."

So Doug begins to pay homage to the long expanse of my boot, beginning at the heel. Moaning with pleasure, he doesn't need much encouragement, but I coo to him anyway. "You're one of the most enthusiastic slaves I've had in my dungeon in a long time."

Suddenly, I feel my slave do something that is quite forbidden. Doug's tongue flicks the bare skin of my thigh. I jump up and push him aside. "You will be punished for that little transgression," I inform him. "Do you know what I do to naughty boys?"

"No, Mistress," he answers obediently.

"I put them over my knee and spank them."

This calls for me to unchain Doug's wrist cuffs. Since I know what it feels like to be chained, I suggest that he shake his arms to restore the flow of blood. "After all, my slaves are my property," I explain further. "I don't want to damage them. They're too much fun to play with."

Although Doug is slim, I feel the full weight of his body as he lies across my lap. Still, I encourage him to wiggle, to squirm. Again, he sighs ecstatically. "Spread your legs so the chains are taut," I say, but not too firmly. I enjoy this almost as much as he does. The outline of his hardening cock carves its shape into my thighs as Doug squirms. I order him to wiggle even more. "The more excited you are, the less painful the spanking will be."

The first smack resounds nicely. His ass cheek jiggles in the wake. I plant the next open-palmed blow on the other side. Slowly, I spank Doug, who thoroughly enjoys each blow with a gasp of pleasure. In between smacks, I caress. And all the while, I sweetly chide him. "You really shouldn't have licked me without permission. You're lucky that you can even go near me."

I pick up the pace, smacking faster now, a bit harder. I know I'm not hurting him, but that he is savoring every swat. The cheeks of Doug's ass are stained a slight pink. I feel my smile grow wider as Doug's moans become more passionate. "Does it hurt, Doug?" I can't help but ask.

"It hurts good, Mistress."

It is time for other things. On his knees before me, I again outline his crotch with the tip of my crop. "I can see you liked that, didn't you?"

"Yes, Mistress."

"But not too much . . ."

"No, Mistress."

"It gets me very hot to see such a good reaction in a slave. Now, you may lick my thigh, this time with my permission. Yes, you do have potential, Doug."

My slave's fantasies run a bit more exotic than a typical cuffing and spanking. He desires to be restrained further, to be whipped, to be tied, to be blindfolded. Since he has hired me to be his Dominatrix for the afternoon, I am more than happy to oblige. I lead Doug to the wooden rack. He stands passively, obediently, as I loop the ropes around his legs, decorating his body with heavy twine. I secure his arms above his head and spread his legs wide apart. "How are you feeling, Doug?" I ask as I mask his eyes with a blindfold.

"Fine, Mistress."

There is one more rope to apply, a thick cord wrapped many times around the waist. Doug sighs deliciously as I fasten the final knot. I run my bright red fingernails down his chest. "Every part of you belongs to me, doesn't it?"

"Yes, Mistress."

Standing back for a moment, I observe my handiwork. "Such a nice, naked body," I tell Doug. "But it still needs a bit of adornment. You don't know what I mean, do you?"

"No, Mistress."

Doug's nipples are hard with excitement. Seeing him bound and helpless before me, I can't resist taking advantage of the situation. I suck on one nipple, then the other, all to the chorus of his groans. Then I bite softly and he moans even louder. "Does it hurt, or does it hurt so good?"

I don't bother to wait for an answer. As I stroke his flesh with a black feather, my appreciative slave whimpers again. "You make the nicest of sounds, Doug," I tell him. "It seems as though you're in slave heaven."

"I love it when you call me 'slave,' Mistress," Doug coos.

"This is only the beginning." Gently, I apply a clamp to each of Doug's nipples and give alternate tugs. His first response is a loud groan, perhaps because he is so unaccustomed to the sharp sensation. "You must learn to take the pleasure with the pain so that pain is pleasure and pleasure is pain," is my advice to him.

I stroke Doug's cock, which I have liberated from the tight briefs. Cupping his balls, I flick at the nipple clamps with my other hand. It is as though slave Doug is in a trance of pleasure/pain. "All my life . . . all my life," he murmurs. And I know exactly what he means. All his life, he's dreamed of this moment. He's fantasized about it, even masturbated to thoughts of domination in the lonely dark. But finally, he is living his fantasy.

"Have you ever been whipped, slave?" I ask.

"No; Mistress."

"I'm going to begin with a soft whip," I explain, holding up one of my favorites. It is thick at the handle and has many tassel-like tendrils. Teasingly, I hold it between the cheeks of his ass. "I wonder how you'd look with a tail . . . maybe you'll be my pony some day!"

Although I was only joking, Doug responds with a hearty, "Anything for my mistress."

I tell Doug to kiss the whip. As I place it against his lips, he does so eagerly, touching it, sucking it into his mouth. It arouses me to watch his total absorption in the act. "Now that you've kissed the whip, I'll let this whip kiss you."

"Please, Mistress! Please whip me!" he cries.

"One day, you'll see the whip marks on your body as little presents from me," I tell him.

First, I let Doug feel the creamy leather streamers against his skin, tickling him. "You've felt my whip's caress, but you haven't felt its sting."

Before I begin, I grasp my slave's scrotum in my fist. "Who has you by the balls?" I ask.

Doug is almost sobbing with pleasure. "My Mistress! Mistress Jacqueline! My beautiful Mistress!"

The whip is poised in the air. "I'm going to give you ten, Doug, and I want you to count. The way you count is to say 'Thank you' after each stroke. One, thank you, Mistress. Two, thank you Mistress."

As my whip kisses slave Doug's back, my mind drifts off. I am vaguely aware of his counting in the distance, but my thoughts are consumed in the duality of this scene. A few years before I was the one in Doug's vulnerable position. I had a need to be punished. I was the submissive, the slave. No, my life wasn't always like this—being in control, having power. All too often, I found myself being the victim, both emotionally and physically.

But now things are different, very different.

2

Alice

My real name is Alice.

In my mid-thirties, as a practicing clinical psychologist, I'm still trying to find out what makes me tick. Many of my early problems with men—including Daniel, my husband of several years—stemmed from the fact that I never dared tell them that deep inside I was a submissive woman. Before I discovered my tendencies as a Dominant, I enjoyed playing the role of "slave." A loving but forceful spanking on my bare bottom brought me to incredible erotic heights.

I live in two worlds. One is as a clinical psychologist with full degree credentials. But, in a bizarre role reversal, men also hire me to help them live out their desires to be submissive. So, in a private dungeon in my own apartment, I become a professional Dominatrix.

When my marriage first dissolved, I tried to escape my awful feelings of inadequacy by using too much alcohol and drugs. Along the road, I've fondled hundreds of cocks and fallen in love many times with the wrong guys for the wrong reasons. Sadly enough, I've never found a man with whom I could totally merge myself. In this feminist era of "take charge" women, I am the personification of that image, as a loving Dominatrix wielding a whip, yet I also had the need to be dominated.

Technically, I should be a pretty little suburban Jewish housewife with two kids and an adoring, if slightly boring and balding husband. But my wheel of fortune landed on another number. As you continue reading the story of my life, perhaps you and I can discover some of the reasons we become the kind of sexual people we are. If you continued to walk down the straight and narrow path you were born on, then why didn't I?

As a professional Dominatrix, I have some of the most influential men in America at my feet paying for my services. There are those who view me as a high-priced or specialized prostitute, although I never engage in sex with my clients. Rather, I help them live out and realize their innermost fantasies and fetishes. In addition, I provide a caring and accepting environment for their hidden secrets and "forbidden" objects of arousal.

I have chosen this job for a number of reasons. First, because I am an intuitive and understanding individual, boasting degrees in both education and psychology. (Because it might be considered unethical, I choose not to use my therapist's license in my line of work.) Second, I choose to be a Dominatrix because I too had a fantasy that I once felt I'd have no choice but to hold inside as a terrible secret for the rest of my life. When I finally "came out of the closet," I felt a sense of extreme relief and great gratitude toward the man who helped me unburden myself. I very much wanted to write this book to help others, to let you know that it's perfectly all right to express yourself in whatever way feels comfortable, even if it appears to be out of society's definition of "normal."

How did I go from being a nice, straight, middle-class Jewish girl to a sought-after Dominatrix? It is a story of emerging self-esteem as well as great change, for as I grew closer to becoming "Mistress Jacqueline," I really began to like myself. As a young woman, I was shy and intimidated by men. As a submissive, I fully enjoyed physical and verbal abuse. And as a Dominatrix, well, you'll soon find out. But first you'll have to get to know Alice.

Alice was born in the Bronx, New York. I grew up in the stagnancy of the late 1950s and the early 1960s in a two-bedroom apartment with my mother, my father, and my sister, Robin. We were a pretty typical, middle-class, Jewish family, not rich, but not poor either. To the outside world, I'm sure ours appeared to be a good home. Robin and I were well-fed and well-dressed, but emotionally our lives were barren.

My father was a hard-working man. He ran his own business and left for work by six or six-thirty every morning, arriving home late

every night. My mother never held a job outside of the home until
I went away to college. She felt very strongly that it was her place
to be home. My mother's incessant doting became another part of
the problem. Robin and I were both pressured into being high-achiev-
ing children. Mom constantly reminded us that we were sent to the
best summer camps, that we had piano lessons, dance lessons, and
all the rest. We did well in school, but somehow it was never good
enough. The piano lessons and camps were fine, but even then I knew
they were only window-dressings. I needed things of more substance.
I needed my mother's affection, her acceptance. I needed her love.

Alice was a very pretty little girl with long, blonde ringlets. Physically, I suppose I was a beautiful child, but somehow I never liked
myself. Even though I had natural blonde hair, somehow I thought
I should have had brown hair like everyone else. Perhaps that was
the problem—I never felt quite like everybody else. My father and
mother never laughed much, never acted silly or seemed to really enjoy
life. They also didn't seem to know how to show affection, except
by providing material things. The words "I love you" were not in their
vocabulary. They never told me, "You're pretty" or "You're smart."
If I scored an eighty-five on a test, it should have been ninety. If I
scored ninety, it should have been ninety-five. I never seemed to be
good enough.

When I was very little, I can remember hugging my mother, putting my arms around her and holding her as tightly as I could. That's
the way I wished she would hold me. But whenever I did that, I recall
her always asking, "Are you sick? What's wrong? Why are you hugging
me?" There always had to be a reason, some excuse, to show love.
Why couldn't I hold her just because I felt like it?

My mother was a fanatical housecleaner. I could never be in her
presence when she performed her chores. I'd be in the way. I'd mess
things up. As a result, I'm very undomestic and barely know how to
sew a button on a shirt. But my mother was Supermom. She did it
all and she didn't want help from anyone.

Although Mom might sound like a refugee from Europe, she's not.
Like me, she was born and bred in the Bronx. My father's family is
from Poland. He was born overseas and came to the United States when
he was five or six. My mother always made it crystal clear that it was
her side of the family that counted—that Dad's side was lower class.

Robin is six years older than I am. I really liked her a lot, but as kids we fought a great deal. I can remember times when her friends visited and they'd often make fun of me. Although I don't remember it, Robin told me that one of her pals went so far as to tie me up as I screamed at the top of my lungs. I don't think my later spanking fantasies stemmed from this, though. Even when I used to play submissive, I wasnever into being tied up.

My mother constantly seemd to be at war with my sister. She often slapped her right in front of me. Watching them, I'd end up sobbing. I never wanted to bring friends home because I was embarrassed that they'd start fighting. One time Robin ran away because Mom wouldn't let her go to the amusement park with her friends. I was so afraid she'd never come back that I cried and threw up all afternoon. Of course, Robin did come back. When I was five or six, I began vomiting a lot. It was an emotional reaction to the unhappiness that surrounded me, almost like bed-wetting is to other kids. I'd even wake up in the middle of the night and tell Mom I was sick. I knew it would make her angry, but I couldn't help it.

I was such a mess that my mother took me to a child psychologist. It is still a very vivid memory for me. I remember going to her office and doing some type of play therapy with her. I was actually having a nice time. Then the therapist told me to leave the room. I overheard her talking to my mother. "There's nothing wrong with Alice," she said. "She'll grow out of this vomiting stage. It's just her way of asking for love and attention." Once Mom heard that I'd be all right, she tuned out the love and attention part. When I told Robin I needed more love, she teased me. "Love and attention, love and attention, the little girl needs love and attention," she used to cry, mockingly.

Although I wasn't a happy child, I did very well in school. I was always at the top of the class. By the age of twelve or so, I was "boy crazy." I'd always pursue the ones who were the most popular, the unattainable ones, the boys *everyone* liked. Of course, I'd never get them. In grade school, it was Paul. He had a crew cut and clear blue eyes. He made it a point to ignore me and I made it a point to pursue him. At summer camp, I was in love again, this time with a guy named Howie. But he didn't know I existed. I never chased the ones I could get, only the ones I couldn't. But I did chase boys—literally. All of us girls would chase the guys, catch them, tie them up, and spank them.

In the sixth grade, my best girlfriend was Barbara. She was the most popular girl in class. We hung around and were always getting into some kind of trouble together. We were even kicked out of the Girl Scouts. But Barbara could be extremely nasty. "You know I'm much prettier than you are," she'd tell me very cooly. "I can get the boys and you can't." Once we dated a couple of boys who were friends. My boyfriend happened to be cuter, but Barbara made it a point to assure me, "You know that will never happen again." I even remember a time when Barbara beat me up and somehow I was blamed for it.

What it all amounted to was I felt bad about myself because of my home life. Naturally, my friends were people who treated me badly. It followed suit. It was something I was comfortable with. My mother never missed the opportunity to tell me that I was a rotten kid. "You're worse than Hitler," I can still hear her shouting. Imagine a mother telling her own child that. What could I have possibly done that was as terrible as a man who had killed millions of human beings? Still, I carried those feelings inside of me even in the outside world.

I'm still not certain where my bondage fantasies evolved from. As a youngster, I can remember rubbing myself against my bedsheets and fantasizing about being spanked. In real life, I was never spanked on the behind, but I certainly was beaten. Thrashed severely. My mother would break wooden hangers on me. She would pelt me with a pipe from the washing machine for even the smallest act of disobedience. Maybe I craved the normalness of being spanked, the sanity of being swatted like a child and not flogged like a plantation slave. I recall playing with my little girlfriends in the park. We'd sometimes spank each other. I suppose it's part of playing games like "house." Spanking is something most mommies have to do, but somehow it also registered as something sexual to me.

I do believe that fetishes start early. As a clinical psychologist, I often see that with my clients. When people have a fixation fetish, where they're fascinated with something like women's feet or legs or by infantilism, those things seem to have started at a very young age. Most people can't even recall when it originated. Some of my clients discuss early childhood experiences of an older sister or aunt who beat them. Experiences like these often lead people to conclude that women are superior. Although I rationally knew that my domination fantasy was a bit bizarre, it was still something that turned me on. As I often tell my S&M clients, as long as your fantasy turns you on, consider yourself lucky to have something that will always arouse you!

In junior high school, I managed to get into something called the

"S.P.'s." It's a special program for smart kids. I remember the debate
Mom and I had about whether I should enter the two- or three-year
program. Ultimately I enrolled in the two-year program. Even though
I got away from some of my "bad seed" elementary school friends,
I found myself gravitating toward the same types of people in junior
high school. You know, the girls who were a little bit bad and a little
bit boy crazy. Of course, I'd get into trouble, because of horsing around
in class or giggling. Typical teenage things. But in my house, you were
in hot water if you were five minutes late for dinner. Imagine the uproar when I'd have to stay late for detention. I hated to provoke my
mother's screaming and yelling, but I couldn't resist being mischievous.

Most of the time, my dad never got involved. He was more of
a peripheral figure, wrapped up in the details of his business. By the
time his work day ended, it was late. He'd have just enough energy
to read the mail, eat dinner, and read the paper. This was his scenario
night after night. If my mother and I happened to be embroiled in
a bitter dispute, he'd halfheartedly try to break it up. Then Mom would
yell at him for trying to break it up. They forever played out the roles
of wimp and domineering bitch. Maybe that's another reason why I
was intrigued by S&M. For me, it was a very normal way of life. I
grew up watching my mother reign supreme over my father. S&M,
however, is only a game. It should be playful and sexually gratifying.
The roles are defined and people aren't really degraded. That's not exactly the way it was between my parents.

Even as a kid I wondered why Dad didn't just slam her, slug her,
and tell her to shut up as he quietly went back to eating his pot roast.
But he never did. My mother emasculated him and perhaps he enjoyed
being subservient to her. After a long day at work, all Dad wanted
to do was sit for a moment and sift through the mail. Mom would
be rushing him along, whining, "Come on, it's late enough. How long
do you expect me to keep dinner warm?" And he'd rush to the dinner table.

I am paid to say the kind of things to men that seemed to come
quite naturally to my mother. Even on car trips, she would degrade Dad
for getting lost. She never ceased to remind him that he wasn't handy
around the house, coming very close to ridiculing him. It was pretty awful
to watch. Today, I realize that I was picking up silent, unfavorable hints
about male/female relationships from watching them. "Men are made
to be pushed around," was the message. Then again, maybe my par-

ents needed each other in a perverse sort of way. Perhaps Dad needed a woman to play "top" (dominant) with him. And that's just what Mom did, and continues to do. Although I don't see them very often, they're still married after all these years.

I saw a different side of my father during an incident that happened when I was a student at Boston University. I came home for a week when Mom was suddenly rushed to the hospital. It was scary at first because we didn't know what was wrong with her. Diagnosed as an ovarian cyst, her condition wasn't life-threatening after all. My first thought was, "At least she'll be out of the house for a while." I kept hoping that my father and I could have a nice time together without her and finally get to know each other.

It didn't turn out that way. My father couldn't function without Mom. Even with me there, he was a lost soul. He'd come back from visiting her at the hospital with lists of instructions. That's the only way he seemd to be able to get by. "Water the plants . . . pick up milk . . . don't forget to pay the electric bill." It was plain that my father felt frightened and uncomfortable at the thought of facing life without Mom. I suppose I did hate her for making him an emotional cripple. Basically, my father is a good man, but I still harbor some anger that he didn't stand up to Mom's rantings, for himself, and for me, too. The few times I confided in him, Dad would run off and tell Mom my secrets.

My folks still live in New York, but they spend winters in Florida. During my last visit home, I began to see them in a different light. Recently I've avoided visits back east, partly because they have no idea how I make a living. I'd like to keep it that way, but still find it difficult to always be weaving a web of lies to tell them.

Because of my nephew's bar mitzvah, I flew home from Los Angeles one January. While I was in town, my father's sister happened to pass away. Mom felt badly, but was anxious to get back to Miami. Sitting shivah (the traditional Jewish period of mourning) for seven days didn't fit into her plans. While Mom was ranting, my father very plainly told her, "Look, if you want to go to Florida so badly, you go. I'm staying here." His "you go your way, I'll go mine" approach shocked her. It was a strong side of him none of us had seen before. I do have to give my mother credit for her response. "Get that out of your mind," she told him. "I don't want you to stay here alone." For the first time in her life, my mother compromised. Because she relented, Dad left a

little earlier than he had originally planned. I was surprised to find myself thinking, "Good for her. She got what she wanted." But it wasn't
by yelling or screaming. It was by giving in just a little bit.

Maybe, in some ways, I've overreacted to my mother. For many
years I was too submissive in my relationships with men. I began to
drink too much and used drugs to blot out the bad feelings I had about
myself. For the past three years, thanks to my involvement with a well-
known drug and alcohol counseling group, I have more control over
my life. I think I've grown up a lot.

But when I was still a child, the seeds of these problems were
planted. When I was ten years old, my sister Robin went out of town
to attend college. As soon as she left, all the fighting and all the household strife became focused on me. I was the sole object of my mother's degradation and beatings. In those days, child abuse wasn't something people discussed openly. There was no one to call. I just suffered through it.

When I was in high school, my mother began beating me with
wooden coat hangers. I'd go to class with welts and bruises on my
arms, but no one ever said a word about them. I recall a very petty
fight about being forbidden to phone a boyfriend. Although my father
was usually the one who broke up the fights, he began to thrash me.
It was the day before New Year's Eve and I had a date the next night.
When I persisted in wanting to call my boyfriend, Phil, my father started
hitting me in the face. Instead of stopping him, my mother joined in.
So there I was, with both of my parents pelting me. I finally shook
them off, but stumbled away with my face swollen and bleeding. En-
raged, I knew there was something called the Child Humane Society.
"I'm going to call them and tell them how you beat me," I screamed
at my father. I don't know if I could have actually done it, but when
my father saw me looking up the telephone number, he had a change
of heart. Dad took me in his arms and told me how sorry he was.
I suppose that was enough—for the moment.

Despite my heated family disputes, I never perceived myself as an
abused child. I came from a nice Jewish family. Nice Jewish families
can't be bad. My parents sent me to summer camp every year. What
they didn't know was that I couldn't wait to get out of the house. A
typical kid, I hated authority figures. I broke tiny rules so I could feel
powerful and just a bit wicked. Nothing too serious, just enough to
get my parents into an uproar.

In camp, I didn't warm up to the counselors. In turn, they were happy to ignore me. I always became friendly with Miss Troublemaker. She'd prod me to play kissing games with the boys and I would gladly agree. Never the ringleader, I was always the willing follower. I would do almost anything to be accepted, to feel a semblance of love.

There's usually at least one positive adult figure in the lives of kids like me. How else could we survive? For me, it was my maternal grandmother. She was very sweet and loving, and, strangely enough, my mother was very close to her even though they were so unlike in temperament. Unfortunately, my grandmother died when I was six. Mom was never quite the same after that. She probably felt abandoned by her mother's death. But instead of growing closer to her daughters, she continued to push Robin and me further away.

Somehow, in junior high, I won the lead in the big school play. For the first time, I was truly happy. Not only did I love myself, but I learned that I loved acting. I was so enthusiastic that I wanted to go to the High School of Performing Arts. (It was popularized by the movie *Fame* and ensuing TV series.) But Mom discouraged me. She thought it was silly. Since I hadn't started at age five like Shirley Temple, it was too late. Of course, I was discouraged, but I listened to my mother.

It's just fairly recently that I have had the courage to start taking acting lessons. Performing and creating a new persona is something I've done in my work as a Dominatrix. After lots of work, I feel I'm a convincing actress. Perhaps you'll agree after watching some of my videotapes or catching a glimpse of me on programs like "The Sally Jessy Raphael Show" and "The Joan Rivers Show." Once again, I proved my mother wrong. If you really want to do something, it's never too late. Never.

I had a girlfriend named Susan in high school. She was very smart, in fact, Susan was brilliant. And she was an overachiever like me. Her family structure was also very similar to mine. Her mother was very dominant, a schoolteacher. Her father owned a novelty shop in the Bronx. Susan's mom was the bright one and never missed the opportunity to bring up that fact. Like me, Susan was driven to perform well academically. She wasn't bad looking, but I suppose she wasn't a beauty queen either. Susan and I became fast friends. We tried to be popular, but were always shot down. Sometimes the "cooler" kids who hung around on the Grand Concourse would make fun of us. They were downright abusive as they attacked our obvious nerdiness. But we'd always come back for more the next week. At least they *noticed* us! Susan and I were an indefatigable team, bravely attending college fraternity parties on Friday nights. Always ignored by the cutest guys, we'd continually strike out. It was pretty awful. Although Susan and I never had a good time at those soirées, we always stuck together. At least we had each other.

Susan taught me the joys of something that ended up becoming a problem—food. Overeating is a very natural Step One for a person who will grow to become a substance abuser later on in life. Yes, Susan taught me the virtues of food. Okay, so maybe there weren't suave college men knocking down our doors, but there were always Hostess Cupcakes to make us feel good. Twinkies healed all wounds. With few guys to divert our attention, we would eat anything in sight. Susan could eat anyone under the table, but never seemed to put on any weight. But by the time I was a high school junior I was lugging around ten or twenty pounds more than I should have been. I wasn't obese, but I certainly wasn't slim. Being overweight added to my horrid self-image. I imagined myself an ugly mess and was convinced that no guy would ever date me. Today, when I look at my picture in the yearbook, I see that I really *was* pretty. The only reason I wasn't popular and didn't have boyfriends was my attitude about myself. I didn't like myself. Very clearly, it showed.

One night Susan and I invited a few of our friends to my apartment. My parents were away for a few days and I was on my own, longing to feel grown up. Our idea was to have a handful of kids attend, but when word got around that we'd have the place to ourselves, people started showing up out of the woodwork. Soon it got out of hand. Beer flowed freely. My mother's carefully waxed kitchen floor was totally scuffed. I was terrified at the way my parents would react. In a frenzy, I tried to kick everyone out. But they turned the tables on me. When I dashed out to get rid of some of the garbage, they slammed the door and locked it behind me. Inside, Susan had to phone her father to rescue us from our own friends.

There wasn't much I could do to clean up. By the time my parents came home, the place was a wreck. Needless to say, my parents were furious. My mother acted as though it was as terrible as the bombing of Hiroshima. I sobbed and told them I was sorry, but deep down I didn't think I had done anything that terrible. They made a tremendous stink about it, though, grounding me for a month. I wasn't permitted to confer with my beloved Susan in person or on the phone.

My parents were very prissy. I never saw either Mom or Dad half-dressed, let alone naked. You had to be fully clothed at all times. Bathroom functions were never stated in words, let alone sexual functions. Belching was a cardinal sin in my house. Once, I was studying for a test in my room, quite comfortable wearing an oversized t-shirt. Mom walked in and gasped, "Cover your thighs! They're so fat and ugly!" If she took me clothes shopping, Mom would tell me I had to wear a girdle. "You can't get away without it," she'd say. "Just look at you."

I did look at myself. For the life of me, I couldn't see what was so awful. As for sex—forget it. My friends and I were properly drilled that sex was one of those things you waited to do *after* you got married. And even then, it wasn't supposed to be too pleasant. Susan and I would giggle and talk about wearing a suit of armor on our wedding night.

The hippie days were just starting. Susan and I fell in with a new crowd that smoked pot, something we'd never tried. The summer before, I'd discovered the luxurious numbing effects of alcohol. My parents had sent me on a cross-country teen tour. Toward the end of the summer, someone got their hands on a bottle of liquor. After taking a few slugs, I began to feel incredibly relaxed. At the age of seventeen, the message that alcohol would loosen me up and give me the courage to be the adventuress I really wanted to be became very clear to me. I admit that Susan and I were nervous about hanging around with a pot-smoking crowd. One night, we finally broke down and tried it. Marijuana wasn't nearly as terrifying as we'd heard. No big deal.

Finally, Susan and I each had a boyfriend in our new circle of friends. Jim was sweet to me, but I was a little afraid of this handsome hippie. He was also into "free love," a concept which also scared me. Everything about love seemed to scare me! By the time I felt ready to sleep with Jim, it was summer and I was already away at camp. So much for procrastination.

When it came time to apply to various colleges, Mom managed to procure a B'nai B'rith handbook that gave the percentages of Jewish men attending particular schools. I was shocked, suddenly understanding the major reason behind her carting me off to school. I was being sent to college for my "MRS" degree, to become a promising, budding Jewish businessman's bride. Women went to college, became schoolteachers, taught for a year or two, got married, had a couple of kids and lived happily ever after. Since I really had no defined goals, I didn't protest too much.

The first year I went off to Boston University, I was elated. I couldn't wait to escape my parents. They knew it, too. Although I could have gone to nearby City College for free and lived at home, I opted to study over two hundred miles away, free from their clutches. My parents didn't have much money, but they probably wanted to get rid of me as much as I wanted to leave.

In the very early 1970s, colleges like Boston University were at the center of student unrest. There were all kinds of academic and political changes shaking the country and the world at that time. Like several million other teens, I had discovered *The Harrad Experiment,* a book about sexual utopia. But Harrad was a far cry from Boston University. At B.U., the dorms were segregated at first and students couldn't even invite guys into their rooms. A few years later, there were open dorms and everyone was fucking everyone else. It was free-love time. Social revolution days. Nobody even bothered with attending classes regularly. We were too busy protesting the war in Vietnam.

Before she shipped me away on my college husband-shopping spree, Mom sternly instructed me, "Don't *ever* let me know that you're dating someone who isn't Jewish. I'll yank you out of school." For more emphasis, she went as far as adding that if I married someone who wasn't of the proper faith, she'd scar my face. When I wondered aloud if she'd prefer me marrying a Jewish street cleaner or a rich, professional gentile I really loved, Mom's response was a sharp, "Don't ask that. You know the answer." With my mother's instructions tucked away in my brain, who do you think my first college boyfriend was? Someone named Brendan McKinney. I felt so guilty about seeing him that we broke up after a few weeks.

I tried to buckle down for one of the most difficult programs at B.U. The courses were ultra-liberal and artsy. We had small classes and frequent discussions. There was a lot of work to do. Because of my new-found freedom, I didn't find it easy to concentrate. There was nobody hanging over my shoulder pushing me to excel.

Protesting the war in Vietnam became the most important item on my agenda, but I also had to maintain my good grades. Because of this, my first two years at B.U. were a turbulent sea of conflict. Although I really wanted to be on my own, I didn't know how to function. Was I like my father? Confused unless someone strong dominated me and told me what to do? There were no special men chasing me. When I wasn't strapped to the textbooks, I smoked dope with my friends and ate a lot. Gaining weight was a good excuse not to deal with men. But in my sophomore year, I fell in love with Jim. I felt very comfortable with his warmth and his nice, big smile. Alone in his room, we'd talk incessantly about the complexities of the universe. He'd hug me a lot. Although I tried to encourage him, it never went any further. At first, I thought he was just shy. Finally, I asked him point blank about it. "I'm a virgin," he said almost apologetically. If he was a virgin like I was, I concluded that he was probably just scared. Still a bit bewildered, I liked him so much that I continued to see him.

Jim told me that he took a bus down to New York City each week to participate in an encounter group. The leader had a theory about people, about how everyone is a certain type of person and how opposites attract. Jim and I were certainly opposites. I was a passionate fool and he seemed oblivious to my desires for physical intimacy. It seemed inevitable that we'd end up making love, but months passed and still nothing sexual happened. Finally, I gathered the courage to confront Jim about our lack of lovemaking. Approaching the subject warily, I tried to be sensitive to his feelings. Unfortunately, Jim wasn't sensitive to mine. "I'm just not attracted to you," he shouted. "All right?" His encounter group had taught him how to express anger, and express it he did, yelling and screaming at me. I just wanted to curl up into a little ball and disappear. Very hurt, I didn't know how to let go. We still spent time together, but he never touched me.

But I was determined to go to bed with Jim. It was crazy. I was in love with a guy who wouldn't make love to me. Finally, I accompanied him to New York and met with his encounter group. Most of the members were at least ten years older than me. They never stopped talking about their feelings, baring their emotions to each other. I liked this because it was confrontational and mentally stimulating. The focus of that meeting was Jim's and my relationship. He admitted that he was still a virgin and had no woman in his life. I was shocked. Sitting right beside him, I obviously didn't count for much. When one of the members asked about me, Jim shrugged. He didn't know what to say.

The group's leader was determined to bring Jim's emotions to the surface. He had us try a "confrontation technique." We yelled a lot, but neither one of us really listened to the other. I was instructed to focus on the wall, think of my mother, get angry, and scream at her. Somehow, I became the center of attention. Everyone asked me how I felt about Jim. Quite plainly, I told them that I really loved him. Jim finally admitted that he loved me, too. The group members insisted that we leave early. Together.

It was late, a misty, moonlit night. We walked down the slick street, but I felt as though I was skimming across a cloud. At last, I was going to make love to a man I really liked and I wasn't afraid. It was almost like a dream. At Jim's apartment in the East Village, we barely looked at each other as we got undressed. I was naked first and suddenly felt very awkward. Jim sat on the side of the bed with a dazed expression on his face. It was as though he had no idea of what to do next. Then he kissed me. I touched him between the legs, but he didn't seem to get aroused. Jim never got an erection that night, no matter what I did or how hard I tried. And I tried everything. Although I didn't really know what I was doing, I put his penis in my mouth. I sucked on it, but he never grew hard enough to enter me. After a while, we just decided to stop trying. You could imagine how badly I felt. From reading *Cosmo,* I knew that you should never confront a man about potency problems. I told him not to worry, that it really didn't matter. We spent the night sleeping in each other's arms, but the atmosphere that morning was very uncomfortable. I went back to Boston and didn't hear from Jim for about a week.

The following Monday, I bused back down to New York to attend the group. Jim was already there when I arrived. Of course, the members were anxious to know what had happened between us. We each told our side of the story. Next, the group leader asked Jim to talk about some of his sexual fantasies. He admitted that he often imagined another guy (not himself) being with a woman. He was a voyeur in his fantasies. The group interpreted this as meaning that Jim might be entertaining homosexual fantasies. Since this was a couples-oriented, heterosexual group, most of them thought that homosexuality was "off the feeling," as they phrased it. They also believed that gay men harbored a lot of hostility toward women. Today, I have a great deal of gay male friends and I know this is untrue.

Poor Jim was so upset that he stormed out of the room. I didn't see him until a week later, when I had the courage to visit him at his apartment. "I don't give a damn about the group," I told him. "What

I really care about is you." My proclamation did no good. Jim was still angry and began shouting at me again. "Nothing will *ever* happen between us," he ranted. "Get out of here!" With that, he grabbed me by the shoulders and shoved me out the door. He slammed it hard behind me. I never saw Jim again. Needless to say, I was still a virgin.

That summer, at the end of my sophomore year, I flew to Israel to visit my sister. Robin had finally married a nice, Jewish boy. She and her husband had decided to live on a kibbutz in Israel. To earn my keep, I held a job there. Although I wanted very much to explore that beautiful country, my main goal was to get laid. I convinced Robin to take me to her gynecologist and I promptly obtained a prescription for birth control pills.

I kissed and cuddled and fondled quite a few guys before it finally happened and even found a steady boyfriend on one of the neighboring kibbutzim. While we were embracing passionately, he tried to enter me a few times. But it hurt so much that he never actually managed to penetrate me. Time and time again, he stabbed his rock-hard penis between my thighs and barely got inside. Technically, I was still a virgin.

Later that summer, I left the kibbutz and decided to see Greece before heading back to the States. On an interisland boat to Mykonos, I met Larry. Surprisingly, he was from Queens. No matter where I went, New York seemed to follow me around. No exotic men, even in exotic locales. But Larry would do.

Back on the mainland, we found ourselves in an erotic clinch high atop a cliff. It was wonderful, but something inside of me was afraid of what was about to happen. I wanted to share my body with a man, but I was still hesitant. Larry's fingers slipped between my legs. I felt myself pushing him away. Still, his hand persisted.

"No," I told him.

Larry was bewildered. "I thought you wanted it."

"I don't know what I want," I admitted. Larry quieted me with a tongue in my mouth. I gave him one big shove.

"One more move like that, Alice, and you'll send the both of us flying off the cliff."

In search of safer surroundings, we waited until we got back to Athens to continue our carnal wrestling match. Lying on cool white sheets, I braced myself for that first fateful thrust. After Larry was inside me and dutifully humping away, I remember thinking, "Is that all it is?"

Larry was booked on a flight back home the next day. Although his family was only a train ride away from mine in the Bronx, he was a student at the University of Michigan. It wasn't exactly a stone's throw from Boston. He phoned me when he was home for the holidays and we did see each other one more time. Another uneventful fuck, nothing more.

Originally, I had entertained the idea of doing my junior year abroad in Israel, but decided against it. One reason was my enthusiasm about the encounter group. I felt it was a place I really belonged.

Every Monday night I took a Greyhound bus from Boston to New York. But once Jim had left, I felt there was no real reason to continue. The other people were much older than I was. You played by their rules or not at all. After one session where I was particularly honest, they agreed that I acted like a bad little girl and needed to get spanked. That struck too close to home! "Do you suppose it showed?" I wondered. Were my spanking fantasies showing through the seams of my well-kept personality? The thought terrified me. I didn't want anyone to discover my secrets. When the other members instructed me to strut around the room like a Mae West–style bad girl, I became so frightened that my hands stiffened up. I couldn't move.

I was attracted to a few men in the group, but nothing ever happened. I even brought Donna, one of my B.U. roommates to a group meeting. Would you believe she ended up meeting a guy she really liked? But not me. Never me. Not only that, but Donna was able to let go of her emotions, get fully involved in the group and do what I couldn't allow myself to do. Although I tried to fight it, I was really jealous. When Donna finally quit college and moved in with her boyfriend, it was too much for me to bear emotionally. My interest in the group waned.

Junior year. I had to decide on a major. It was 1974 and everyone was still letting their hair down. We didn't think of the future. The warring world might blow itself up any day, and then revolution would come. Who could think of the future—or declaring a major? I was sure that if I graduated from college, everything would somehow take care of itself. The same lackadaisical attitude that's been haunting me most of my life. Most of my friends were focusing on liberal arts. That seemed to best personify the atmosphere of the early seventies—morally liberal and socially artsy. I had planned to major in English, but suddenly realized it wouldn't leave me with any definite career choice. So, I ended up doing what my parents had drilled into my brain for so many years. I focused on "elementary education." It was a nice, safe, respectable career choice. "My daughter Alice, the teacher." I'm sure the words had a pleasant ring to their ears. "She can't do much, but at least she can teach."

Although I knew it would please them, I was almost embarrassed about my decision. So traditional, it certainly wasn't "cool." It wasn't like joining the Peace Corps and helping build shanties in Bangladesh. But as it turned out, I enjoyed my education curriculum more than I did the liberal arts fare. Finally, Alice was doing something concrete.

In my senior year I became a student teacher. I worked in one of the nicest districts in suburban Boston, in a town called Lincoln. The school was beautiful and clean, the students well-behaved. In the autumn we'd go out to the surrounding meadows and pick apples with the kids. A pretty picture, something out of *The Corn Is Green* or *The Prime of Miss Jean Brodie*. I felt fulfilled and motivated—so much so that I went to summer school, enabling me to graduate in January.

Immediately following graduation, Mom and Dad wanted me to come home and live with them. They'd support me and put me through graduate school, but only if it was in New York. Life was always a double-edged sword with them—full of complications, little deals, compromises. Since I'd had a taste of freedom, there was no way I could go back to their brick fortress in the Bronx. I made the decision to live on my own. Needless to say, my parents were not happy.

It wasn't long before I would find out that teaching jobs were few and far between. During the mid-seventies there was a mysterious oversupply of fresh-faced instructors like me. To survive as I continued my search I began taking temporary office work assignments. I had done this to earn extra money for the past few summers and during school breaks. (Anything to avoid going home for a visit!) But it didn't help my ego when I realized that I'd sweated through four years of Boston University only to rely on my marginal typing skills. I finally secured a permanent job—as a receptionist. At University Hospital (affiliated with Boston University) I enjoyed working with the cancer patients but I hated the fact that my BS wasn't being put to use.

My self-esteem was taking another blow, but my love life did seem hopeful. I became involved with a medical student interning at the hospital. Richie didn't have the air of a future doctor. Despite his white lab coat, he could have easily passed for a construction worker. Towering above me at almost six feet tall, he had long, scraggly, dark hair and narrow, green eyes. A bit unkempt but kind of sexy. His background wasn't anything like mine. Richie came from a poor family, but I admired the fact that he had single-handedly put himself through medical school.

After a couple of months, I finally realized that Richie wasn't Jewish. Of course, I hid that news item from my parents. In many ways, he was the classic type of guy I got involved with—very consumed with himself and his own interests. If he wanted to go fishing for the weekend, he wouldn't ask how I felt about the venture. I'd be dragged along, sitting on the shoreline, extremely bored but glad to be with him just the same.

More than having a boyfriend, I wanted a career I could feel good about. I felt degraded answering telephones with my fancy college degree. Still scouting around for teaching jobs, I was often discouraged. Only five feet tall, I looked very young for my age. Interviewers often told me that they didn't think I could handle a class of unruly kids. There were always mountains of other people applying for the very same teaching slot. Stacks of other résumés always reminded me there was a lot of competition in my chosen field. Why would anyone in their right mind choose me?

I soon quit the receptionist position and did occasional substitute teaching. With some temp work I managed to get by. Since I shared an apartment with two other girls, I was just able to pay my part of the bills. I began testing the job market outside of the Boston area, going as far as Vermont and New Hampshire. I was both thrilled and confused when I was offered a job four hours outside of Boston in the heart of ski country. "Don't worry, I'll visit you," Richie told me encouragingly. But deep down, I knew I couldn't live there. Not only wasn't I fond of the bitter cold, but I'm too klutzy to even consider taking up skiing. I was certain I'd be bored to death.

Another option presented itself when Betty, a friend of one of my roommates, visited us one weekend. Betty had just landed a teaching job in St. Croix, the Virgin Islands. It certainly sounded more exotic—and warmer—than a tiny town in Vermont. The pages of an old *National Geographic* confirmed that it was a beautiful place. Betty was certain there were more openings and encouraged me to apply by mail.

I did, but soon forgot about this prospect and became immersed in life's day-to-day problems.

Like my relationship with Richie. You might say we'd reached a comfortable rut. Richie lived in a public health service hospital nearby. The pattern was that he would pick me up after he finished work, around ten or eleven at night, and I'd spend the night with him. We had a good sex life. In fact, Richie was the first man I actually climaxed with. He assured me right away that since he was a medical student, he was very familiar with all of those wonderful nooks and crannies in a woman's body. His deft surgeon's fingers would go to work between my thighs, find my clitoris and soon have me quivering and moaning.

I had just discovered the pleasures of orgasming with myself. Nice girls didn't touch themselves "down there," and I was no exception. I managed to work my way around that taboo and still have sensual tremors. Positioning myself beneath the steady stream of water from my bathtub's faucet, I would spread my legs as wide as I could. The relentless flow would bubble over my mound like a tireless brook. I would watch my clit bobbing under the pressure. Then I would close my eyes, my mind taking over at that point. I would fantasize about someone spanking me, dominating me, and very soon I would be shuddering in an intense orgasm.

About the same time, I read a letter in *Penthouse*'s "Forum" section that tickled my erotic fancy. It described a paddling session in great detail. Recalling that passage never ceased to get me off as I furiously fingered my clit. Between Richie's polished diddling technique and my own fantasies, I never had trouble reaching an orgasm. Even though I was sexually fulfilled, I kept wondering why I was haunted by those spanking fantasies. Why couldn't I think about something "normal," like being made love to on a moonlit beach? Isn't that supposed to arouse every woman?

All I knew is that I imagined having my ass swatted by a firm hand whenever I masturbated or fucked—and I always managed to reach a climax. Why was that so wrong? I was drawn to the kinky classified ads I saw in newspapers like the *Boston Phoenix* or the *Real Paper*. I'll never forget one man's ad, which read, "Have you been a bad girl? I'll spank you soundly and soothe you tenderly." With two fingers buried in my warm, wet cunt, I'd whisper that phrase to myself over and over again, fully aroused by the sound of the words, by the way they hung in the still air. But after an intense orgasm, I always felt guilty. Why couldn't Alice be like everyone else? You really are a freak.

Although our sex life was satisfying, Richie and I didn't have much in common outside of bed. In a group, he was always outgoing and funny, the guy who made everyone laugh. I kept wishing he'd be a little more attentive to me and my needs. When it came to men, I was still pretty naive. So terrified of being as dominant as my mother was with my father, I rarely voiced so much as an opinion. I sure as hell didn't want to be like Mom. I was even more certain that I didn't want a wimp like my father as a mate. What I did was go to the other extreme. I became the emotionally abused one. I went along passively with whatever my man wanted. Happy or not, I enjoyed being a martyr. It was the sort of treatment I expected, thought I deserved, and felt comfortable with. A perfect victim. This is around the time I was raped.

3

Attack

I was raped on May 8, a few days before my twenty-second birthday. My substitute teaching was often done in schools located in the middle of a ghetto and I had to deal with a roomful of disobedient kids. It didn't matter what grade they gave you. Second graders tended to be even worse than fifth or sixth graders.

I usually saw Richie every night. One particular evening, he wasn't feeling well and asked me to take a cab to his place. I told him I didn't feel like it. I didn't want to, but guilt about not seeing Richie made me change my mind. Rather than take a cab, I decided to walk the mile or so to his place. It was a pretty spring evening. My route took me through a dark side street near Commonwealth Avenue, a major thoroughfare in Boston, very busy and full of life. Strolling along, I was enjoying the clean smell of the season and the balmy breeze. I was toasty-comfortable in my maroon ski jacket, not looking particularly sexy. Approaching a quieter residential zone, I noticed a big black man following close behind me. We were alone on an empty street. He looked lost, peering at numbers on the buildings. For a moment, I almost turned around and asked if he needed help.

I continued to walk, but was beginning to feel a bit uncomfortable. Now I was sure the guy was following me. Things my mother had told me about being careful skimmed through my head. When I approached the corner, I had to make a turn into the hospital's side street. I wondered if I should call Richie and tell him I was on my way. After all, he didn't know I was coming by. I decided against it, and started to walk faster. Out of the corner of my eye, I saw that the black man had flagged down a car. Relieved, I thought he was finally going to stop following me.

But something just didn't feel right. I could taste fear, cold and steely in my mouth. I started to run toward the hospital door. The man ran after me and grabbed me around the neck. I screamed. "Shut up!" he snarled at me. I'm sure somebody must have heard me struggling to get away, but it was too late. He dragged me into the car. I suddenly realized that it had been trailing us all along.

"Oh, shit! I can't fucking believe this!" I kept telling myself. Inside the car, the driver, another black guy, yelled at me to stop screaming or they'd kill me. I could see his mouth moving, but was so terrified that his words made no sense. The guy who'd grabbed me forced my head down against the back seat's musty vinyl.

"Shut the fuck up," he warned. "If you scream again we'll cut up your face."

The driver was now skidding the car down Commonwealth Avenue like a maniac. I prayed that the police would see him. The awful thing was that I knew no one would report me missing. My roommates assumed that I was with Richie. And Richie wouldn't know I'd changed my mind and decided to spend the night with him. No one was going to miss me. I envisioned being driven to a remote spot. The men would rape me and kill me. In a few days, someone would discover a faceless, nameless, naked body amidst the maples. I kept hearing my mother's constant warnings, "If you're not careful, Alice, they're going to find your dead body someday."

My captor was feeling me up in the back seat. I couldn't tell where we were headed as the other man tore recklessly along. Fifteen minutes later, we screeched to a stop on a dimly lit street in the Roxbury ghetto area of Boston. Dragging me out of the car, the guys grabbed my arms. "Don't bother to scream, Whitey, because nobody's going to give a shit about you in this neighborhood." I saw a couple of black guys. They laughed at my cries for help.

Inside an apartment building, they rang a doorbell, but nobody answered. My rapists had a problem—a victim, but nowhere to take her. Back on the street, a prisoner between them, we walked and walked. I felt my legs collapse under me, but they pulled me up by the armpits. The guy who had dragged me to the car yanked me down on the curb beside him while the other guy left. It turned out he was looking for a place where they could fuck me.

Staring at me with big, belligerent eyes, my original captor offered me a cigarette. It was really bizarre, because for a few moments, we sat there smoking silently like old friends. When I begged him to let me go, he just ignored me. We just started talking. He was much younger than me. I asked if he went to school. "Yeah. Boston High," he said. It was a place where I had often done substitute teaching.

"We won't hurt you," he said in a soft voice. "Just do whatever we tell you."

There I was, sitting on this curb with my attacker. He was big, well over six feet tall, and wore a studded earring. This was way before it had become a fashion statement for men. Later, I told the police detective that it was his only distinguishing feature. The other guy was much meaner. Small. Feisty. He was nasty to me.

Puffing on the cigarette he gave me, I tried to appear much calmer than I actually was. "My boyfriend's expecting me," I told him matter-of-factly. "He's going to start looking for me."

"Don't worry," he assured me. "We'll get you out of here real soon." God, he sounded like a hairdresser soothing a customer who'd been kept waiting too long.

A few minutes later, the guy's friend came back. Whenever he was around, my original attacker became nastier. Walking between them again, I was really frightened. They finally stopped in a dark space between two buildings. I wasn't sure what they wanted. Sobbing, I begged them to let me go.

"Take off your clothes," the mean one snapped, tearing off my jacket.

In total shock, I pulled my blouse over my head. "All the way," one of them snarled. I unzipped my jeans and they fell down around my ankles. Then came my bra and panties. I was naked and helpless in the middle of a concrete alleyway. One of them found a broken cardboard box and forced me down on it. I don't remember who fucked me first. All I remember is a black cock sticking up in the air and one of them climbing on top of me. Pumping violently into my vagina, he climaxed within a few seconds. Then the other mounted me. I kept praying that they only wanted to screw me, not kill me.

I'd been reading *The Happy Hooker* by Xaviera Hollander. I was amazed at how liberated she was. Xaviera could probably fuck anybody. She could probably even cooperate with thugs like these guys. To survive, I tried to put myself into Xaviera's mindset. It wasn't really me. I was a hooker. I was having sex with men I didn't particularly like, but it would be over soon. I even went so far as to pretend that I was enjoying it. It wasn't really that bad. All they did was screw me.

I didn't fight. I just lay back and spread my legs. I moaned and groaned and acted as though I were enjoying it.

"You liked it, didn't you, bitch?" the nasty one said. "Tell us how much you liked it."

"Yeah. I loved it," I told them bitterly.

"Do you want some more?"

"Please. No more," I begged. "I've had enough."

"Why don't you give us your phone number?" said the other. "We could get together again."

I didn't answer. They watched me get dressed. I couldn't find my purse in the dark. "Whitey, you're so careless," they scolded. They kept calling me "Whitey" and lighting matches to help me find my pocketbook.

For some reason, I was stupid enough to ask if they'd give me a ride home. Of course, they didn't. Believe it or not, they did help me hail a cab. They said I could get hurt in a neighborhood like this.

I had the taxi take me to the hospital and I called Richie immediately. He came right down. After the examination he wanted me to go to the police. I didn't want to. Richie said I had to, and eventually I gave in. I gave my report and then Richie and I went with a cop to see if my attackers were still around. We went back to where I was raped and drove around for a long time, but they were long gone. One of the cops cracked, "I wish some girl would rape me some day." He and Richie had a good laugh—can you believe it? My description did eventually help them find the pair, but only after they attacked two other women. I suppose I was lucky, because one woman was forced to do anal sex with them.

Richie was not what I would call supportive when we got back to my apartment hours later. He insisted on having sex with me that night. I really didn't want to, but he insisted. "I just want to make sure I can still fuck you after two black guys did." I went along with it, like I always did.

Psychologically, I couldn't deal with my rape. I wanted to forget the sick fear in my guts as they pounded themselves into my body.

I suppressed my emotions. I even blamed myself. Why hadn't I been more careful? Why didn't I fight harder? I had been too neglectful, too stupid. For a while, I was very afraid of black men, which was ironic, because soon I began teaching in the Virgin Islands. Fortunately, the sexual aspects of being raped haven't been traumatic. I still like men and still enjoy sex. I think of my attack as a bad quick fuck, an unfortunate one-night stand.

It was many years later, when I was working for the Rape Response Program at Cedars Sinai Hospital, that I realized the full impact the rape had had on me. Besides staffing the telephone hotline, we were often sent to hospital emergency rooms to help victims immediately after an attack. We accompanied them to court for their trials. The head of the program stressed the importance of individual counseling, but I felt group situations helped the emotions surface more effectively. The women didn't feel so alone. I was given permission to start Cedar Sinai's first rape encounter group. The only requirement was that the members weren't "in crisis"—that the rape had occurred at least six months before. As a former victim, it was an incredible experience for me.

At the court preliminaries for the trial, my rapists packed the room with their friends. When I tried to explain to the lawyers what had happened, the guys all started laughing. By the time the actual trial came up, I had settled in the Virgin Islands. Later on, I heard that my attackers were each given twelve-year jail terms. Actually, I felt pretty indifferent about it, probably because I've always had trouble with our criminal justice system. When you cart someone off to jail, you often make them worse. If they're rapists when they go in, they may be killers when they're released. I'd much rather have seen my attackers get therapy.

I've never been a vindictive person. What those men did to me was wrong, but I lived through it. I lived. I survived. No big deal. Maybe it's the wrong kind of attitude to have, but that's the way today.

4

Daniel

Richie and I were at a stalemate. I was waiting for him to either ask me to marry him or, at the very least, to move in with him. Neither thought probably crossed his mind, since he roomed with some friends immediately after medical school. Alice was left on the outside looking in once again.

I hadn't had a vacation in quite some time and decided I needed a break, from Richie, from life, from everything. To my amazement, I was offered the teaching position in St. Croix. Before I could accept, I thought I should explore the island a bit. Like a brave little girl, I hopped onto an airplane all by myself. It was late June or early July, just after the height of the tourist season. I immediately found the island residents very friendly. When I told the lady at the tourist information booth that I was researching a teaching job, she introduced me to a friend who worked at a local hotel. He took me out to dinner that night with a jolly group of people. There I was, in a strange place, dancing and drinking with strangers and having the time of my life. Thanks to Richie, I had been getting high on alcohol on a regular basis. That was one of the things we liked to do together. It made me loose, free, relaxed. I felt I could do anything I wanted. Here, in the warm, tropical climate, I was often very thirsty. Those big, sweet drinks with funny names seemed to melt me in all the right places.

St. Croix seemed very quiet, but pretty. For the next few days, I made it a point to do nothing of great importance. Wandering up and down the beach, I relished the sensation of the hot sand between my toes, the sun toasting my skin. There was a group of people my own age hanging around the wharf. Quite boldly, I approached their boat and introduced myself. Open and friendly, they soon invited me to stay at their house. My bags were sloppily packed in a matter of moments and I checked out of the hotel. Sailing was the most serious item on our agenda. I had never seen water so blue. We'd skim across it in the breeze for hours, drinking rum and whatever else we could find. This paradise seemed even more lovely through heavy, drunken eyelids. I had a brief fling with one of my new housemates. My friends introduced me to some of the many Americans who had settled on the island. Bev and Irv from New York ran a seashell shop right on the wharf. Bev introduced me to Annie, another woman who was planning to start teaching on the island that autumn. We decided to become roommates if I decided to accept my teaching offer.

Yes, drinking helped me conquer my fears and shyness. It also helped me blot out things I didn't want to hear. One story I didn't want to hear was about a recent murder case—five American golfers had been gunned down by Rastafarians on the very posh Fountain Valley golf course, which was owned by the Rockefellers. It was out and out murder. Famed attorney William Kunstler seemed to have an affinity for political cases of this sort and was defending the accused murderers. I had heard whispers of racial problems on the island, but tried to ignore them. St. Croix was so gorgeous, the people so warm, how could the rumors be true? When I have my mind set on something, I only see what I want to see. And what I saw was a tropical heaven, a place to party where I could have friends and teach at the same time. That was good enough for me.

Originally, I had planned to stay in St. Croix for only a few days. I wound up extending it to two weeks. When Richie picked me up at Logan Airport, he didn't seem too thrilled. Surprised at how good I looked, he held in his anger about the fact that I'd chosen to accept the teaching job in the Virgin Islands. It was clear that he wanted to be the one to make all the decisions in our relationship.

Of course, my parents weren't happy with my leaving the country, but they no longer had a hold on me. To bolster my confidence, I phoned Betty and asked what she thought about St. Croix's racial tension and the recent murders. She told me not to worry. In fact, she was going back down there to teach herself. Betty offered to share her apartment with me, but I'd already made plans to stay with Annie.

With my mind firmly made up, there were only a couple of weeks to pack my life into cardboard boxes. The night before I left, Richie came by to help me get ready. Almost immediately, we became immersed in an ugly argument.

"How can you do this?" Richie wanted to know. His green eyes, as dangerous as broken glass, took me apart.

"Do what?" I asked, calmly folding a sweater against my chest.

That was it. Richie hurled a box across the room. The clothing I'd neatly folded rained down upon the floor. Silently, I gathered the garments up as Richie screamed and yelled, bashing my suitcases around with his feet. Although he didn't hit me, Richie certainly demonstrated a lot of violence toward me. Only a few months after being raped, I was witnessing yet another violent man in my life. I couldn't wait to leave.

In St. Croix everything seemed to fall into place. Annie and I flew down together. The first thing we did was buy a car to get around the island. It was only twenty-eight miles long. The man who sold us the car knew of an apartment available in a housing development nearby. That afternoon the landlord showed us around a pretty duplex townhouse, complete with two bedrooms and two baths. Annie and I felt as though we were in a whirlwind. We couldn't make a decision between us, so the landlord poured us each a huge drink. After only a few sips, everything seemed clear. We signed the lease. There was even a week or two to relax before the school term began.

The St. Croix school system was very different than what I was used to back in the States. As a student teacher in Boston I'd worked in the best, most progressive schools and in ghetto institutions, too. But I wasn't ready for anything as backward as St. Croix's teaching system. There was very little in the way of resources and reading materials. We had to practically fight for textbooks. The major thing the administration liked you to do was to keep the kids quiet. There were two types of teachers. The Cruzan teachers were black island natives. Then there were people like Annie and myself, the imported white breed. The resentment toward us was obvious. "Continental" teachers is the respectful term they'd call us. It was the one they used to our faces, but we knew we were most often referred to as "honky" teachers. As a rule we were given the worst classes and had to work in the most terrible conditions.

I must have been lucky, because I was awarded a group of fifth graders, the exact age group I'd wanted. It was a 5-2 class (5-1 being the smartest) and was composed of bright, eager students. I took a liking to them right away and as a result worked hard to prepare intellectually stimulating exercises for them. The first few weeks I was up until eleven most nights working on lesson plans. I was very happy to finally be teaching.

A steady stream of letters began to flow down from Boston. Richie. He swore again and again that if I hadn't left he would have married me immediately. I had to laugh. Had I blown it yet another time?

Island life was very much like that in a very small town. Since there were only two bars in the area, patrons got to know each other like family. Everyone would be in them on Friday and Saturday nights, drinking their souls into oblivion. During the week, it was work. On weekends, it was sailing excursions. It seemed that nothing could disturb this pleasant, partying existence. But then something went wrong. Something always goes wrong.

I'd only been in St. Croix a few months when a white Frenchman was killed in one of the bars we frequented, "The Gallows." Frenchie supposedly asked for a brand of beer they didn't carry. Harsh words were exchanged and later he was found murdered. It was definitely a racial attack. I was afraid.

The very next day, two female continental teachers were reported missing. Soon their bodies were found washed up on the beach. One of the victims was Betty, the very one who had assured me about the safety of St. Croix. This hit too close to home. If I'd been Betty's roommate, would I have been the bloated, lifeless body next to hers?

The exact details surrounding the double murder were never disclosed, but the homey climate of the island changed drastically. Everyone became wary of everyone else. The Fountain Valley Golf Course murders had slowed down tourism considerably, but this new turn of events brought it to a grinding halt. Life on St. Croix very quickly sunk almost to poverty level. Even the most established hotels were closing their doors. A number of teachers decided to leave. I would have left too, except that I loved teaching so much. Going back to the States might mean never standing in front of a class again, never seeing children brighten when they discover something intriguing. I couldn't abandon that. I'd finally discovered something I was good at.

Richie had some vacation time in October and came down to visit me. This was right after the murders and he kept trying to convince me to hop on a plane with him. One night, we were lying quietly in bed. "You're next," he whispered into my ear. "They're going to get you next. It happened to you once. It will happen again." I turned away from him and pretended to be asleep.

I was glad I'd decided to at least finish up the school year in St. Croix. My students were very loving toward me. Although they were poor, and although there wasn't much hope for their futures, I really felt as though I was making a difference in their lives. We learned together and I felt like a vital part of the universe.

Alcohol was very plentiful on St. Croix. When you ordered a Screwdriver, it was three-quarters vodka and just a splash of orange juice. Needless to say, it didn't cost much to become an alcoholic there. Every day after classes I would drink. St. Patrick's Day was a holiday the natives especially loved to celebrate. Kids as well as adults would drink unabashedly in the streets. Besides drinking, drugs weren't difficult to find. I had a prescription for Quaaludes, pills I especially enjoyed because they made me feel more sexual. Marijuana had that effect on me as well, and it was very easy to find, too. I didn't analyze my chemical indulgences too deeply. All I knew was that drugs helped me become the uninhibited woman I craved to be. The partier. Beautiful, exotic Alice. This Alice was wild. This Alice wasn't afraid of men. She wasn't afraid of anything, except maybe herself.

Men were numerous as sugar cane, and I had a sweet tooth, fucking every guy in sight. Soon I fell for another schoolteacher, Mark. Things were pretty good between us at first, but then he pulled away from me. Whenever a man does that, I tend to want him even more. Mark was a very handsome Vietnam veteran. He had a rough edge to his personality and I never felt I could penetrate to what lay beneath his skin. For a relationship of the flesh, I suppose I was satisfied. Mark's best friend, Wayne, also lived on the island. Wayne's lady, Jane, was also a schoolteacher, so the four of us had fun bouncing around St. Croix.

Mark was the first man I ever admitted my spanking desires to. He caught me off guard, suddenly asking if I had any sexual fantasies. Bracing myself, I tried to tell him, red-faced and almost choking out the words. He was unimpressed. "Oh, no," he said. "I have to do that to the kids at school all the time. I'm tired of using my belt. What else?" There *was* nothing else. That was my dreaded secret and I'd finally shared it with someone—unfortunately, someone who didn't understand.

Our relationship quickly became stale but that never stopped me. Around Carnival time, I accepted his half-hearted invitation to accompany him and Wayne to a friend's house on nearby St. Thomas. Since sleeping quarters were limited, I found myself sharing a bed with the both of them. Mark instructed me to stroke his friend's cock. Despite feeling guilty about my friend Jane, I did. The three of us made love that night. I kept both of them happy with my hands, mouth, and pussy. It was exciting, despite my inhibitions. I liked the feeling of two sets of hands caressing my body. Afterward, I drifted off to sleep, feeling like I was a very sexually liberated person.

When I woke the next morning, I expected all of us to be the best of buddies. But Mark was distant and left unexpectedly for St. Croix two hours later, leaving me alone with Wayne. He tried to get friendly, but I was unresponsive. Quite frankly, I didn't go for his type of lovemaking. He was too rough in all the wrong places. Despite Mark's lack of interest in me, I still wanted him. I seemed to desire most what I couldn't have.

After Mark, I was back to my *Looking for Mr. Goodbar* existence. That seemed to be another thing I was very good at—drinking until I could barely stand and picking up men who were bad for me. Amazingly, I was able to keep up with my daytime responsibilities at the school. My teaching won me favorable evaluations and I got on famously with Mr. Salinsky, the principal.

I spent most of that summer in New York, but couldn't wait to get back to St. Croix to teach the following September. Looking up old high school friends, I phoned Ellen. We giggled about old times and filled in the blanks of recent years. A budding yenta, she seemed to know who was doing what and where. "You wouldn't believe who I saw," Ellen told me. "I just ran into Daniel Fidel, and he looks incredible."

I hadn't seen Daniel in at least five years. We had been good friends in high school. He played class clown and I laughed at his jokes. The last time I'd seen him, he wasn't much taller than I was. At sixteen, he looked like a kid of twelve. We had even gone on a few dates, but I quickly discovered that he wasn't my type. Older-looking guys, college fare, turned me on. I had seen Daniel one more time when

I was home on a sophomore break. He'd helped stage a mini-reunion of Roosevelt High's graduating class. We all met at the "Alice in Wonderland" statue in Central Park at a designated time. It had been two years since I had seen Daniel, and I was shocked. Not only had he grown almost a foot, but he was very handsome. We dated a few more times and he even took the bus to Boston to pay me a visit. I didn't go to bed with him because I was sleeping with Richie at the time. That Christmas break, Daniel took me to a Laura Nyro concert and we planned to spend New Year's Eve together. Because he wasn't feeling well, Daniel didn't want to go out that night, but asked me to come to his apartment. I made some unintentionally flippant remark like, "I guess I'm just not worth spending money on." Daniel didn't say anything. He just slammed down the phone. I never heard from him again and kept trying to tell myself that it didn't matter.

Talking about Daniel on the telephone with Ellen, those old feelings surged back. It seemed they were mutual. Daniel had even given Ellen a letter to forward to me in St. Croix, but, of course, dizzy Ellen had forgotten to do it. She fished it out of one of the messy heaps I knew littered her room and read it to me. Daniel certainly had a way with words. His letter was a very funny, upbeat description of his experiences in college and his cross-country travels. He ended it by stressing how much he wanted to talk to me. I phoned him immediately, happy to hear his warm, friendly voice. He seemed glad to hear mine, too. We made plans to see each other on July 4th.

Meanwhile, I had somehow managed to keep Richie hanging from a string the whole year I'd been teaching in St. Croix. I knew I had to break up with him, but I was never good at doing that kind of thing. I was more comfortable being the one who was dumped on, not the one who caused the hurt. I had left a lot of possessions in Richie's apartment and he threatened to throw them out unless I came to Boston. As a result, I had to break the date with Daniel, but he seemed to understand.

It was an uncomfortable confrontation. Amid all of Richie's ranting, I managed to gather up my belongings and leave. Happy to be on a bus again, I headed toward my sister and brother-in-law's place in New Jersey. They had cashed in on kibbutz life and were full-fledged suburbanites. Robin was kind enough not to tell my parents that I was still in town. Immediately after I settled down, I learned that Robin and Bob were about to spend a week in San Francisco. While I was free to tag along, I wanted to see Daniel again. I couldn't stop think-ing about the guy. Even though nothing serious had developed, there was something about him that I really liked.

A few days later I found myself wandering through Greenwich Village, seeking out the address I'd hastily scribbled down on a scrap of paper. It was a nice building facing Washington Square Park. Stand-ing in the elevator alone, I didn't quite know what to expect but my heart was thumping hard. I'll never forget the way Daniel looked at me, hungrily, surprised. "God," he muttered, "you look great." Tanned to a golden brown from being in the Virgin Islands, the globes of my breasts were bursting out of my halter top. I was a little heavier than I am now, but Daniel insisted that he liked me better zaftig. I was glad Daniel Fidel found me very sexy.

He had a whole day of activities planned for us. Unlike "dates" with Richie, our time together wasn't going to revolve around getting drunk. In fact, Daniel didn't drink at all. We took a walk on the West Side Highway, which was closed for reconstruction at the time. Dan-iel had even packed some sandwiches so we could have a little picnic on the concrete. We talked and talked a lot, somehow getting into a discussion of those titillating *Penthouse* letters. At that time, the two major fetishes were amputees and spanking. We laughed about the most outrageous entries as we walked along, admiring how pretty the Hud-son River looked over our shoulders. Of course, I didn't let on what an arousing effect those spanking letters had on me. At least Mom and Dad would be happy that I finally found a nice, Jewish man I really liked. Since Daniel and I had practically grown up together, conversation flowed very easily between us. He managed to keep me laughing and smiling all day long. After all of the nasty shit that Richie and I were constantly hurling at each other, it was a breath of fresh air. We passed a small bar where the Nitty Gritty Dirt Band would be playing later that night. Daniel picked up tickets and took me out for savory Chinese food.

I ached to spend the night with Daniel after the show, but I didn't dare tell him. It was getting late and I kept saying that I had to check the bus schedule so I could get back to New Jersey. He didn't answer. For a moment I was afraid he didn't want to sleep with me. Daniel just watched me nurse a rum and coke, not even having a drink him-self. The alcohol made me feel a bit looser. Back at his apartment, we went out onto the terrace to watch the city's lights. Daniel took me into his arms and kissed me. At that point I knew I wasn't going back to New Jersey.

I felt very vulnerable making love with Daniel at first, more so than with anyone else. Silently we watched each other strip in the dim room. It felt odd taking my clothes off in front of him, maybe because we'd known each other for so many years. It felt odd and vulnerable, but it also felt very good. It felt comfortable, like home. Our lovemaking wasn't what you'd call passionate, but I sensed that Daniel cared about me. By the gentle way his fingertips caressed my nipples, so delicately, as though he were afraid they might break. Wrapping my legs around him, feeling him softly rock inside of me was the most warm, secure sensation I've ever experienced. Of course, I fell madly in love with him. Right now, tears are coming to my eyes because I've always loved Daniel so much. The story doesn't have a happy ending.

After that night, Daniel and I spent much of the summer together. My sister Robin's place became my home base, but I practically lived in Daniel's apartment. I'd call my parents from pay phones and pretend I was traveling around the country. Actually, I was just a short subway ride away, but if they knew I was in town they'd break this lovely spell. Not only would I have to stand up to their barrage of questions, but I would have to live by their rules. I could do nothing right in their eyes. But everything felt so right when I was with Daniel. This way, I had complete freedom. It was the first time I had been able to enjoy New York without having to account for my time.

During the summer Daniel and I took a side trip, hitchhiking to the Rocky Mountains. We had planned to camp out but it was raining most of the time. We ran into all kinds of people—leftover hippies living off the land, growing their own vegetables and marijuana, and poor families who had lived in the stark mountain towns for generations. Everything seemed beautiful. I was in love and smiling all the time, sure that I loved Daniel more than I had ever loved anybody. We'd talk for hours about life, about the past. Daniel was very understanding, especially about my breakup with Richie. I told him everything, especially about how he was always wounding my fragile ego. Daniel, on the other hand, was always trying to build up my self-esteem. "Just be good to yourself," Daniel would say. "Go out and buy yourself a present."

Like me, Daniel was a teacher but couldn't find a decent full-time job in the States. Instead, he worked as a paraprofessional at Hughes High School, one of the worst institutions in Manhattan. He taught remedial reading. At night he worked at New York University's computer center. Since his mother had worked at NYU for years, she'd been able to get him that nice high-rise apartment in the Washington Square Village complex. It was a dreamlike summer. We'd laugh and make love. We'd visit all of the local comedy clubs, something Daniel loved. He often said how he dreamed of being a comedian one day.

Just before Daniel and I became involved, he had ended a relationship with a beautiful, blonde WASP named Martha, the type of girlfriend that seems to drive Jewish men crazy, the kind of woman their mothers always warn them to stay away from. Daniel seemed to take great delight in telling me how pretty Martha was and what a flat belly she'd had. "If you lost ten pounds, you could look like that too," he kept reminding me. "But you'd look much better than she ever did," he'd throw in for good measure. Almost overnight, I became a fanatic exerciser and a borderline anorexic. I wanted to become perfect for Daniel.

More than anything, I wanted Daniel to ask me to move in with him, but he didn't. To complicate things even more, a woman he'd met in his travels was on her way in from California and planned to stay with him. Nothing serious. Platonic, you understand. I cringed to think of this faceless Valerie sharing the small studio apartment with a man I loved. Even though it was difficult, I gave Daniel the space to be with her for a few days. My sister Robin kept telling me not to get angry, and I didn't. There was nothing I could do about it. I was trying my best not to force our relationship. Daniel and I were pretty honest about our feelings for each other. We kept saying things like, "I love everything about you," or "I'm crazy about you." But we were always very cautious not to say, "I love you." Daniel knew that I was planning to go back to St. Croix in September. I kept trying to find a teaching job in New York City, but it was nearly impossible. Before I left, I couldn't avoid spending a few days with my parents. Painful as they were, I lied about my departure date so I could spend a week with Daniel in the Village undisturbed. Our time together was over in a flash. Although I couldn't bear to leave him, I did.

After a tearful goodbye at the airport, I called Daniel the night I arrived in St. Croix. He told me he was lonely for me already. "Alice," he pleaded. "Take a plane back right now. Come home." Home. Did

I finally have a home? Was it by Daniel's side? Is that what he was trying to tell me? It was a tempting thought to leave right then and there, but I didn't. I kept hoping that he'd decide to try for a teaching job in St. Croix, but he didn't even consider it. Daniel was a confirmed New Yorker. He claimed that he couldn't imagine living anywhere else. In the meantime, I was being faithful to Daniel amid a tempting, tropical paradise. I didn't have any dates and I didn't want anyone else. Since there was little else to do in St. Croix except drink and fuck, I was growing a bit bored.

The year before, I had been incredibly attached to my students. They say that every teacher finds her first class very special. It took a bit of time to warm up to my new crop of kids. Nothing seemed the same as it had been the year before. All I could think of was being with Daniel. To complicate scholastic matters even more, the assistant principal of the school had been promoted to principal. Miss Jenkins was a big, black Cruzan lady renowned for her ugly temper. She and I never got along, even before her promotion. As time went on, her aloof manner became more of a problem. She made it difficult for me to get even the most fundamental school supplies. Whenever I was late she scowled at me like a disgruntled bear. I was literally on her shit list. She kept a log of teachers' latenesses and other minor transgressions as though they really carried weight in the crumbling island school system. I suppose I was looking for reasons to leave my job because I just didn't feel comfortable being there anymore.

Luckily, Daniel flew down for a visit during the Thanksgiving holidays. Despite my hopes, Daniel didn't like St. Croix as much as I did. My daydreams of him falling in love with the tropics, deciding to teach there and living happily ever after disappeared like water into hot sand. Daniel craved the excitement of Manhattan, the clubs and restaurants, seeing the latest movies as soon as they were released. He was stricken immediately with what we call "island fever." He couldn't wait to get back to civilization. Even our sex left much to be desired. It was not the sweaty, sweltering kind of encounter on moon-drenched nights that you might imagine. It was just . . . okay. Nothing special. But at that moment it didn't register that anything could be wrong with Daniel. No. It just seemed that things were wrong with us in the islands.

The night before Daniel left, I really tied one on. I suppose that's the only way I could deal with him leaving. After a hung-over farewell at the airport that Monday morning, I drove to my school, unenthusiastic about starting classes again. And late again. It was starting to become a habit, but I really didn't care. As one of Miss Jenkins's prime tardy offenders, I was escorted to her office for another stern talking to. I wasn't in the mood for that. Not this morning.

Miss Jenkins wasn't in yet, but her infernal late list was. There it sat in plain view on her desk. I'd always been curious about what she really wrote down on it, and here was my chance to take a peek. As luck would have it, ill-humored Miss Jenkins happened to walk in just as I was taking a look at her precious late list. To say she overreacted would be an understatement. She went completely berserk, accusing me of "rifling" her desk and stealing things. That's all I needed, especially when I was feeling delicate and wounded by Daniel's departure. Picturing myself as very abandoned and very alone, I burst into tears. Somehow, I managed to pull myself together and get through my classes that day.

A few days later there was a letter in my mailbox informing me that Miss Jenkins had decided to cite me. Apparently "rifling" of desks wasn't proper behavior in the Virgin Islands. She'd taken the liberty of sending a copy of the document to my supervisor, as well as other key people within the school system. I was frightened as well as angry and helpless. Although I had no proof, I hadn't touched anything in her private domain. I'd only snuck a peek at her silly late list. My friend Jane suggested that I sue for "defamation of character." Crazily, I went ahead with a lawsuit. After that, teaching and seeing Miss Jenkins every day became almost impossible.

At Christmas I flew home and stayed in Daniel's apartment. This turned out to be a disappointment. He wasn't very loving, certainly not as attentive as I'd needed after my ego-bashing episode with Miss Jenkins. All Daniel seemed interested in was watching football on TV. Sobbing, I told him I couldn't go back to St. Croix. (Like a good girl, I probably waited until halftime before having an emotional breakdown.) I guess this put him on the spot about our living arrangements. I didn't want to get an apartment alone, so Daniel suggested I move in with him. Our target date was February 14, Valentine's Day.

To make my visit even more complicated, Daniel was having terrible stomach problems. He was plagued with diarrhea the entire week. The longer I stayed, the sicker he became. Of course, this put a damper on our sex life, but making love wasn't a top priority for me. I just wanted to be with Daniel, to sleep beside him, to feel his warmth in the night. I also wanted him to feel better, but when the time came for me to head back to the Virgin Islands, Daniel's condition took a turn for the worse.

I shouldn't have even gone back to St. Croix, but the truth is that whenever I have to make an important decision, I get confused. I would rather stay in a bad situation than make a change. But my friend Jane decided to leave, too, and by February I was ready to leave, just as Daniel and I had planned. I made it a point to send a long letter explaining my side of the story to the local newspaper. To my surprise, they printed my tale of woe.

Right before I left St. Croix I learned that Daniel's bad stomach had evolved into a case of colitis. He was dehydrated and had lost a great deal of weight. He had to be hospitalized. Because he was so sick, Daniel's parents picked me up at the airport. I hadn't even told my own folks about my decision to leave the Virgin Islands—or, of course, to move in with Daniel. I figured I'd break it to them once I arrived.

I was fond of Daniel's parents. The first time I met them, over the summer, I was very nervous. "Daniel's so good," I remember thinking, "they're going to wonder what he's doing with someone like me." There was no reason in the world for me to feel like that, but my self-esteem was scraping bottom. The only thing that saved me was my little vial of Quaaludes. Careful that Daniel couldn't see, I chewed off a tiny piece of a pill right before going to meet them. It calmed me down considerably. In those days, I needed drugs or booze to give me confidence. Meeting them at the airport was a bit awkward. I didn't even know where I was going to stay. Almost reading my mind, his father said that Daniel suggested I stay at his apartment. Relieved, I asked if they could take me to see Daniel at the hospital right away. His mom seemed amused that I cared for him so much. "Of course, dear," she smiled. "Where else would we take you?"

In the sterile hospital hallway, they tried to prepare me for what I would see. "Don't expect anything," Daniel's father warned sweetly. "Daniel's a bad patient. He's been very sick. Now that he's getting better, he's complaining and throwing things around." When I saw what Daniel looked like, I couldn't believe it. He seemed lost in the huge hospital bed, he was so thin. Intravenous tubes jutted out of one arm. When his parents left us alone, it was almost like a scene out of *Love*

Story. I crawled into the bed beside him and held him as tight as I could. So happy to finally be with him, I couldn't stop crying. Nothing mattered anymore because I had Daniel. That's what Mom and Dad had taught me. Once you meet a man that you love, everything else magically works out.

While Daniel was in the hospital, I had his apartment all to myself. Visiting him every day, I wasn't even concerned about finding a job. Even though I was a long way from the tropics, in the middle of a typical, dreary, New York February, I didn't care. This was exactly where I wanted to be. But when Daniel finally came home, things weren't as perfect as I'd hoped. Still run down from his illness, he was in a terrible humor. To make it seem more like home, I stuck a poster of mine up on one wall. The first thing he did when he walked into the apartment was tear it down. Perhaps he resented me leaving my mark so soon after my arrival. I ignored this little performance. Other grating fragments of Daniel's personality became apparent, but I ignored them too. I tried to be forgiving, knowing that he was sick and in a lousy mood. At the same time, I wished he wouldn't view me as an intruder, but as an ally, someone who loved him.

Whenever Daniel made a suggestion, it was like listening to an oracle. The voice of God had spoken. One day, he said, "Don't you think it's about time you got a job?" It was a little too blunt. I was hurt, but I went to an employment agency the very next day. I accepted the first offer that came along. It was with a Japanese firm at the World Trade Center. It wasn't the kind of job I wanted, but I took it simply because Daniel thought I should work. I could handle office work, but I hated it. The Japanese tend to treat their female employees like second-class citizens. One of my responsibilities was to serve the male executives during their coffee breaks. Gritting my teeth, I did. Since I'm chronically late, the time clock became my enemy. If I punched in at 9:10, I tried to make up for it by ending my day at 5:10. I figured there was no problem with that since I had still put in an eight-hour day. But this didn't fit in with the ceremonious rules and regulations. "No, no," the head honcho kept trying to tell me. "Must have excuse. Say anything. Say elevator stuck. Say train late." I tried to comply, but I wasn't very good about being clocked, regulated, and modified. I lasted only three months.

When I was working, my relationship with Daniel was more placid. It wasn't as exciting as it once had been, but we slowly adjusted to living together and had only occasional tiffs. During arguments, he often did the cruelest thing—he would totally ignore me. One time, at a Patti Smith concert, he refused to talk to me until I begged for his forgiveness. It's a behavior pattern he learned from his own parents, because his father often did the same thing to his mom—just as I learned to be the scapegoat, the victim, from watching the way my mother treated my father.

Although I knew very little about S&M at the time, when I think of it now, I thrived on being submissive to Daniel. I was the "bottom" and he was the "top," as the terminology goes. We weren't physically acting out those roles. He wasn't whipping me or tying me up, but the emotional aspects of an S&M relationship were there. Daniel insisted that I enjoyed it when he was ill. Maybe he was right. When he was healthy, he was very independent. But when he came home from the hospital, it was the only time he allowed me to take care of him, to serve him.

I enjoyed parties, being with lots of people. I liked drinking, drinking anything. I wasn't particular. Daniel wouldn't even take a sip of wine. Sweet or not, he didn't like the taste. Very soon I began doing enough drinking for the two of us. Daniel liked to go to bed early, so I developed the habit of getting half-crocked as he slept peacefully, only a few feet away from me. Soon, I'd be blitzed enough to crawl into bed and drift off to jumbled dreams.

On Saturday afternoons, Daniel would play softball with his friends. In fact, he often did things alone with his male friends. I didn't have many friends, so I wound up being home a lot. Either that, or I tagged along. Daniel played baseball. Alice watched Daniel play baseball. Daniel watched baseball on television at home. I wasn't allowed to talk to him during ball games, just during the commercials, so I'd just sit beside him, sometimes sipping wine, sometimes not. Most of the time I was just happy to be with him.

A month after I moved into Daniel's apartment, I finally called my parents and told them I was no longer in the Virgin Islands. They remembered Daniel from high school. I admitted I'd been seeing him, but not that we were living together. How could I? They never liked him very much, and besides that, I knew there would be hysterics if they discovered that their daughter was "living in sin." It was difficult living a double life in the same city as my parents.

One day I broke down and told them the truth. Daniel and I had fallen in love. We were living together to make sure it was right to get married. I don't remember exactly what Mom said, but her voice pierced my brain through the telephone wires. "You must have gone crazy," she screamed. My parents believed in sex only after marriage. I'm sure they decided I was nothing but a whore. In the confusion, I must have blurted out my address before I hung up the phone. Two days later, I received an elaborate typewritten letter from my mother. (At the time, she was working as a secretary at Lehman College in the Bronx, and as a result had gotten very formal and businesslike.) She wrote in detail about how devastated she was and how totally horrified my father felt. Of all people, he wanted to think of me as his virgin daughter. This was the early seventies. How could I tell them that most young people weren't virgins anymore? Didn't they read the papers? Along with the letter, Mom also compiled a neat, two-column comparison (also typewritten) that weighed the pros and cons of living together versus getting married. If you lived together and had a fight, one of you could just pick up and leave. But married people had no choice but to work out their problems. When two people lived together, the family couldn't care less. But when you got married, there's a wedding. People buy you gifts (i.e., a bedroom set that she and my father were trying to bribe us with—an entry which really made Daniel and me laugh). The comparisons went on and on, the next one even sillier than the one before.

Then, one fateful Saturday afternoon, the doorbell rang. I opened the door to see my father standing there. Had Dad dared defy my mother and come visit the prodigal daughter alone? (I later found out he hadn't.) He seemed impressed with our large studio apartment, complete with a balcony and downstairs doorman. I tried to tell him how happy I was and that everything was all right. Daniel assured him that he loved me and told him that we would get married soon. When I rode with him downstairs in the elevator, Dad's only comment was, "At least you're living in a clean place." That was it. There was no understanding and no acceptance of Daniel.

A few weeks later, my father had a heart attack. Of course, Mom blamed it on me. Throughout his life, Dad had a high cholesterol problem along with a heart condition. But the heart attack was entirely my fault. Thankfully, he survived. The major thing I learned about "the Daniel incident" was that I couldn't tell my family the truth about anything ever again.

As Daniel and I settled into "marriage" without benefit of a rabbi, Daniel's parents decided to move into an apartment building right next door. I wasn't too happy about being close to them at first, largely because of the way I felt about my own parents. But Daniel's folks were entirely different. It didn't seem to matter to them whether we were married or not. For the first time in my life, I felt as though I really had a family—a normal family that wasn't always screaming. Daniel's mother was very warm and loving. In some ways she reminded me of my grandmother, the only person who ever told me I was good or pretty. And Daniel's father was always ready to give me a big, warm hug. He managed a clothing store on the Lower East Side and often brought things home for me. They lavished gifts on me and were more interested in what I was doing than even Daniel was. It became a tradition to have Sunday night dinners with them, after which they'd pack the leftovers for us to take home.

I finally had a bonafide loving family. Not only did I love Daniel's parents, but I loved his cousins, aunts, uncles, and even his grandmother. Daniel's brother Harry and his wife Marlo were hardcore hippies who lived a simple existence in Denver. Daniel's parents weren't happy that Marlo had decided not to have any kids. Daniel was very positive that when we got married, we'd have a family. After all, married people had children. That's the way it was. Daniel had very strong, black-and-white feelings about some things and that was one of them. I didn't have any overwhelming maternal instincts, but I thought they would come in time. Right now we were worried about simple things like paying the rent and having a few extra pleasures in life. Having children was the last thing on my mind. All I really wanted was to be in love, and I certainly was.

Around that time, many of Daniel's friends were getting married. Weekends were spent attending other people's weddings. After one celebration, we decided not to go home to Manhattan, but stayed with some friends in Yonkers. A heap of blankets on the floor suited us just fine. In the midst of making love on the carpet, Daniel gazed into my eyes. "Alice, will you marry me?" he asked. "I really love you." Would I? I couldn't hold back the tears. My dream had finally come true.

That was in April. We decided to get married the following June. The year progressed smoothly. Daniel's mother got me a secretarial job at NYU's School of Dentistry, with good benefits. It wasn't at the main campus, which was practically outside our door, but way uptown. They soon discovered that I wasn't a very talented secretary, and I was demoted to doing shitty, menial work. Still not functioning well in the nine-to-five format, I stayed on because Daniel and I needed my paycheck. Daniel wasn't very happy teaching remedial reading at Hughes High School. Most of his students could barely read, and it was a violent, scary place besides. Finally, Daniel agreed with me. "Let's get the hell out of here," he said.

The both of us went to work trying to figure out a place where we could get good teaching jobs. I was veering toward a warm climate. Arizona, maybe. But Daniel had something else in mind. He wanted to go to Denver, where his brother Harry lived. The thought of cold winters didn't thrill me, but Daniel made most of our decisions. I had very little say in what we did. Although he applied to the Denver public school system and received a somewhat promising response, there was nothing definite.

In the meantime, we were embroiled in the complexities of making wedding plans. My parents wanted us to have a traditional Jewish affair at the same catering hall where my sister Robin had been married. Daniel and I wanted a simple outdoor ceremony. But since my parents were footing the bill, they thought they should get their way. Daniel's parents thought that since it was our wedding, we should have exactly what we wanted. Of course, that put them on the outs with my folks. Daniel and I found one place in Connecticut that was absolutely gorgeous. The ceremony would have taken place on a lush, green hill, but besides being too expensive, we could only have forty guests present. My parents wanted a big fiasco where they could invite all of their friends and show off. My idea of a wedding was totally different —an intimate outdoor celebration, perhaps with some wine and cheese. Mom was appalled. She and Dad wanted a big, schmaltzy mess. The very thought of it appalled me. Then there was the insanity of shopping for a wedding gown. Since I felt that getting married was a special, once-in-a-lifetime occasion, I decided to look in Saks Fifth Avenue. Immediately I saw a simple dress with an Empire waist and a splash of lace on the top. Since I'm so small, I'm traditionally difficult to fit, but this dress fit perfectly. Even though it was Saks, I didn't think the price was outrageous. I was so excited that I'd found the perfect wedding gown, I couldn't wait for my mother to see it.

Of course, Mom thought Saks was too good for me. She insisted on taking me to a wholesale house on Broadway. One Saturday I relented and went gown-shopping with my mom. I think a bride-to-be should be pampered and that's certainly the way they treated you at Saks. Like you were special. But this wholesale house was about as special as a fish market. Women were dashing here and there, grabbing gowns off racks. The shop manager kept clapping her hands to get our attention and shouting above the din. I couldn't concentrate. I couldn't find anything suitable. Just as it had been when I was a kid, my mother kept picking out the most hideous outfits, trying to convince me that I liked them. Mom also kept stressing that I couldn't get a white dress. Obviously I was (gasp) no longer a virgin. Another entry in her tearful, typewritten letter stressed that people would laugh and snicker if a woman of questionable virtue dared to wear white at her wedding. Daniel said, "Fuck it. Wear white anyway. We'll just hand out 'Snickers' candy bars to encourage them." That's one thing I loved about Daniel. He could always make me laugh, even in the most hopeless situations. And being with my mom in the wholesale house was certainly hopeless.

A headache was creeping up my neck, nestling between my eyes. I didn't have the strength to argue with her, so I stuck to the off-white restrictions she imposed on me. But those homely gowns she chose for her less-than-perfect daughter struck a sore spot that ran deep. I was ten years old again. I wasn't pretty. I wasn't much of anything. And obviously, I didn't deserve pretty things. Somehow, I made it out of there in one piece without strangling my mother or hurling myself out a window. Since I was still working at the time, I decided to save up the money and buy my own wedding dress—at Saks Fifth Avenue.

We had made our engagement announcement in June, so my parents kept nagging us to get married in December. But Daniel and I had our hearts set on an outdoor wedding. We hung on until June. All of us finally ended up making a compromise. We would set up a tent in Robin's back yard in Fairlawn, New Jersey, hire a rabbi, cater in food and drinks. It was fun helping with the wedding preparations, as long as it didn't involve arguing. I helped choose the menu and select the colors for the tablecloths, napkins, and, of course, the yarmulkes.

Daniel had never bought me an engagement ring, a fact that probably greatly irritated my mother. But I didn't care. Jewelry didn't mean much to me at the time. It seemed trivial and materialistic. "Who cares about diamonds?" I thought. All I wanted was Daniel. Instead of spending money on an elaborate mantilla, I decided to wear a garland of flowers in my hair. But at the last minute Daniel's parents decided to get me a headpiece to match my gown, as a birthday gift. That was more than my parents had offered. In fact, throughout the wedding I couldn't help feeling that Daniel's mother was more mom to me than my own. The day of my wedding, my mother immediately went to discuss details with the caterer. I was left to fend for myself. It was Daniel's mother who helped me put on my gown and wrestle with the headpiece. My mother was more concerned about the hors d'oeuvres than her daughter. It wasn't the first time I felt abandoned by her, and wouldn't be the last.

The night before the wedding my parents insisted that I sleep at their apartment. I'm sure Mom secretly hoped that my hymen would grow back miraculously and I'd be virtuous by morning. What could I do? I had to spend the night with them. Daniel and his father drove me back to the Bronx, making all kinds of jokes along the way. I was depressed, even a bit terrified, at the thought of being trapped there with my parents. We watched the eleven o'clock news in silence. When the weatherman mentioned a chance of rain the next day, Mom glared at me. "See? What did I tell you?" No loving feelings were exchanged between the three of us that night. My parents weren't making this wedding for me. They were doing it to impress their friends and relatives.

The sun was shining in the morning. It was a confused jumble, getting dressed, taking pictures, greeting guests. I felt confused and lost, but the moment I saw Daniel, I felt safe and secure. I ran over and kissed him, so happy that he would soon be my husband. Daniel was nervous, but my assurance put his mind at ease. I was so sure we'd go on happily ever after. I certainly didn't think it would crumble a short six years later.

But on my wedding day things seemed perfect. To calm my jitters, I had a few drinks and was visibly tipsy when I walked down the aisle. The rabbi didn't know us from a hole in the wall. He had our names scribbled down on a scrap of paper, which he kept glancing at. He was so nervous himself that he kept mixing words up. He said stupid things that were supposed to be profound. "The words 'united' and 'untied,'" he growled, "have only one juxtaposed letter. And one letter can make all the difference." Daniel and I couldn't help looking at each other and grinning, careful not to burst into hysterics.

Afterward, I was "celebrating" a bit too much, indulging in more than my share of champagne. At one point, my Dad pulled me aside. "For God's sake, Alice. Eat something!"

"I don't need food," I stammered. "I'm just so happy."

5

Wife

Daniel and I decided not to spend money on a honeymoon since we were planning to leave New York for good in a couple of weeks. We went back to his apartment, now legally "our" apartment, I suppose. Suddenly I was having an alcoholic letdown from the stagnant heat of the room and a sick feeling in my stomach from all of the drinking. I felt strange. All of a sudden, I was married. All of a sudden, things were different. The ring felt heavy on my finger. Our matching bands were made of three bamboo strips of gold. Mine felt uncomfortable, too tight. Everything was closing in around me.

Daniel and I sat on the floor and counted our money. People had obviously taken his "no bonds, only money" hints to heart. Somehow, being married didn't seem as romantic as I'd hoped. I remember feeling that very profoundly. Now that we had society's permission to fuck, some of the forbidden thrill was gone. The permanence, the reality of belonging to each other, felt very odd. In the coming weeks, we would analyze our friends' marriages, always arriving at the same conclusion. Ours was the best. It wasn't just sex. There was a deep element of friendship between us. And we weren't the typical newlyweds, squirreling away money for a house and kids. We were out for adventure. We didn't give a damn about china patterns or color schemes. Who gave a fuck if our bathroom towels matched? We were thrill-seekers about to leave New York to find our fortunes.

We left for Denver about three weeks after the wedding. Since Harry and Marlo were out of town, we had their house all to ourselves. I quickly discovered that this wasn't the place of my dreams. It was sort of ancient, without most of the modern conveniences found in a typical suburban home. I suppose I was caught up in my own trip. I wanted to be a free spirit, but I still wanted everything neat and traditional. Rustic junk didn't fit into my scheme of things. Even though the house was in the heart of downtown Denver, we weren't too comfortable getting around. Harry left us their old car, but since Daniel didn't drive at all and I wasn't adept at operating a stick shift, we took buses and walked. Compared to New York City, Denver seemed hickish. It wasn't the pretty place I'd expected. Daniel, however, thought it was great. I just laughed and said, "It's the ugliest city I've ever seen," trying to make light of it. But Daniel didn't think it was very funny.

"What the hell did you expect?"

I didn't expect anything.

"It's always the same. Nothing's ever good enough for you, Alice!"

Hearing him scream at me like that made me cry. It was our first married people's fight. Daniel just didn't understand how frightened I felt in that strange, forboding city. We had a little money, but no jobs. We were all alone in a place I didn't want to be, hadn't chosen to be. I didn't know what the future held.

Neither of us had any luck landing a teaching job. We'd met a few people, but no one we could connect with or imagine as genuine friends. After a hopeless, wandering week, Daniel asked if I wanted to leave Denver. His parents were paying rent on our New York apartment for a few months, just in case we decided to come back. We could head back east, or try our luck further west. Both of us loved San Francisco. We were sure work in our chosen fields would be difficult to find there, but we decided to go for it. We quickly closed the savings accounts we had just opened and left for a foggy city full of strangers.

Except for my cousin Glen. Like me, Glen was a black sheep of the family. He made a living distributing "Nancy's Yogurt" up and down the Coast. I thought he was a fun person to be with and hoped that he and Daniel would like each other, but they didn't. Daniel thought Glen was a spaced-out druggie/hippie. In turn, Glen couldn't tolerate Daniel's arrogance. He'd gone to California to escape that kind of attitude.

Our first night in San Francisco was spent in a threadbare hotel.

The next day we found a nicer place with weekly rates. Although we weren't living in the lap of luxury, my fond memories about the city were confirmed. Pretty, very different from Denver. Wine was sold openly in all of the grocery stores. I liked that a lot.

When we'd left New York, frozen yogurt was just becoming popular, but in San Francisco no one was selling it yet. The possibilities equaled dollar signs in our minds. Sitting in Golden Gate Park one day, we happened to meet a young couple named Kyle and Maureen. From the heart of the Midwest, they belonged to an odd religious order, the kind of people I didn't think Daniel would want to spend a minute with. But there he was, spilling our frozen yogurt moneymaking idea to virtual strangers. Daniel wanted Kyle and Maureen as partners in the scheme, so we became very friendly with them. Somehow I never did feel comfortable with them—they were always talking about the complexities of the cosmos and their curious spiritual group. We spent a lot of time together in the next few weeks researching the yogurt idea. Since my cousin Glen was in the regular yogurt business, he had access to all of the machinery necessary to make it. Daniel and I even tried to get a small business loan. But with our luck, a big outfit named Johnston's was ready to burst on the scene with the same idea. They were a virtual corporate giant with money and marketing behind them. Without financial backing, Daniel and I had to sit back and watch someone else profit from our wonderful idea.

Despite that major disappointment, we decided to stay in San Francisco. We told Daniel's parents to start shipping our belongings out to the apartment we'd found on Pine Street. Right off Fillmore, it was a small apartment complex with very reasonable rent. There were a lot of young people in the building. Our next-door neighbor was a Cleveland native named Lena. Since Daniel still didn't like to drink, Lena and I would often guzzle jugs of wine together. Daniel soon found baseball buddies and I gathered a circle of drinking companions. During the day, Lena and I would look for work, but at night it seemed that everyone in the complex would gather to drink and talk. I'm sure Daniel must have felt left out, but he never said anything.

Next on the agenda was figuring out how we were going to pay our bills. I'm cursed with being resourceful and responsible, almost to a fault. Throughout our marriage, Daniel always relied on the fact that I could easily secure a humdrum job and bear with it, just so we could eat. Within a couple of weeks I was a perky receptionist at Glassman

International, a firm that sold building supplies to architects. It wasn't too thrilling, but it was something. Daniel decided to take his sweet, old time to find a job he really liked. It was a pattern that continued all through our marriage. I was always working and he was always looking for his dream job. The only problem was that he had no idea what it was. With his diverse background, he could have easily gotten a computer job, but that didn't appeal to him.

The reason I loved teaching so much was that I liked making some sort of visible contribution, helping people, getting immediate emotional gratification from the students I worked with. I found none of that being a receptionist. Answering telephones didn't satisfy my needs. I was just a pretty girl at the front desk, that's all. I couldn't help but be resentful toward Daniel. I was working at a job I didn't like and he was taking it easy. Finally, very pissed off, I told him that *I'd* find a job for him. Grabbing the classifieds section, I read him a perfect ad. "How would you like to manage property for a real estate firm?" I asked him. It turned out to be a decent position, and Daniel was hired immediately. Even though he had never held an office job before, Daniel actually seemed to enjoy it. For the first time in those early weeks, I actually felt as though we had some kind of future together.

While we were in San Francisco, practically all of our New York friends came to visit us. We must have gone to Fisherman's Wharf a million and one times. Another favorite spot was a big comedy club called "The Holy City Zoo." I kept encouraging Daniel to give it a try, but he kept making excuses. His colitis would act up if he got nervous onstage. He wouldn't be very good. Etcetera. I knew his stories well. Leaving the Holy City Zoo with a visiting friend, Ben, Daniel immediately burst into his "I know I can do standup" spiel. Apparently, Daniel had written some long-forgotten comedy routines back in college, and Ben prodded him to dig them out of the archives. Ben suggested that they polish up the skits and get Daniel ready for amateur night the next week.

I was glad Daniel was finally going to test out his dream, but he'd recently gotten laid off and I expected him to be diligently searching for another job. I was off at work while he and Ben laughed and clowned around, sprucing up his few minutes in the spotlight.

As the time on the appointed day grew near, Daniel began to get cold feet, but Ben kept his ego primed enough to get him onstage. I must admit that it was exciting. I was filled with the wonderously scary feeling that something big was going to happen, that an important change was about to take place in our lives. Very nervous about his debut, Daniel didn't eat a thing all day. He arrived early at the club, put his name in a hat and waited to be called at random. His five-minute comedy routine was churning through his brain until he finally stumbled onto the stage at midnight. He was so fatigued from not eating that he practically fell down. Daniel's performance wasn't spellbinding, but he had a few good lines and managed to get some hearty laughs out of the crowd. His nervousness was painfully visible, and as he stepped down from the stage, I hoped that he'd gotten the comedian out of his system so that we could buckle down and focus on the real world. On the way home, Daniel and Ben kept reliving Daniel's moment in the spotlight, talking about it to each other. I was excluded from the conversation. Any comments I made seemed to get Daniel angry. Perhaps I was too stupid to understand the complexities of comedy.

"You were fine," I told Daniel. "But if you never do it again, that's all right with me, too."

Daniel glared at me. "From now on, comedy is my life," he informed me bluntly. He had made his decision, and I was not a part of it.

From that day on I was Daniel's paycheck. It wasn't my choice. I didn't enjoy supporting a struggling artist or having a husband determined to break into show business. That had never been part of our plans. Ben extended his stay another week so they could work up more material. The next amateur night, Daniel's performance was more relaxed. He still wasn't a knockout, but he was much improved. Daniel soon discovered that the comedy circle in San Francisco was awfully cliquish, but he was determined and started spending a lot of time at the best comedy clubs. He decided to enter a week-long comedy competition even though he would be competing against people who had been doing the circuit for years and probably muttered their routines in their sleep. To be different from all the others, Daniel offered a new routine every night. Although his delivery could have been better, his material was good. It was easy to see that his real talents were in writing, not performing. He had plenty of satiric topical comments to liven up his act. All in all, the competition was a good experience for Daniel. He met a lot of people, including Bobby, who is now a very well-known working comedian. He also met Dana Carvey, who won the competition. Dana went on to become the Church Lady on "Saturday Night Live" many years later.

Accompanying Daniel to the competition every night, I was only a peripheral figure. I felt as though I didn't belong in this circle of funny, witty people. After all, it wasn't my career choice. I know I wasn't very supportive, but I suppose that deep down I had fears that our love was on the line. So early in our marriage we were already growing apart. Daniel had turned his life around and didn't seem to care whether I was for or against his new choices. Most of my negative feelings probably stemmed from my insecurity. There he was, out late at night in the spotlight surrounded by attractive women—more attractive than me, I was sure of that. While I'd be dutifully working standard office hours, he'd be doing the night shift at smoky clubs. Today, I know myself better. I realize that I was really just jealous of Daniel, of his courage to do what he wanted in life. Being an exhibitionist, *I* wanted to be the center of attention. It silently killed me seeing Daniel getting all of that recognition night after night. On top of that, I was trapped in a monotonous day job to support his new obsession. Did Alice have any dreams? Did Alice have any hidden talents? She was too busy trying to make a living to realize it.

San Francisco was very much a sexually open town. There were strip clubs and gay bars all over. Publications for swingers and other sensual adventurers flooded the newsstands. In fact, gay people could openly enjoy their lifestyles without being made to feel peculiar. I liked that. I liked the danger, the sense of wildness, the freedom. Flipping through the "want" ads, I couldn't help skimming through the notices for strippers and dancers. The thought always intrigued me. Did I dare undulate my hips and peel off scanty clothing in front of a roomful of anxious men? Would they desire me? Would they get hard for me as I bumped and gyrated to sultry music? Me? Little Alice? Yeah, right.

Not only was the idea alluring, but so was the salary. You could easily make $1,000 a week by showing your nipples to strangers. It all seemed so easy, much easier than answering telephones for seven hours a day, five days a week. I craved something I could be good at. Immediate reaction, immediate gratification, just like the applause Daniel received at the comedy clubs. But I had to laugh at myself. Little Alice making men hot and seethe with desire. Really, Alice.

There was also an interesting phenomenon called "encounter bars." They were places where you worked in a small glass booth and talked dirty to men while they stroked themselves. They paid you just for the privilege of looking at your bare flesh and to hear your words. I don't know, maybe you spread open your pussy so they could see. Maybe you had to play with yourself, too. I was always good at that. I was very good at making myself cum, as long as I had my spanking fantasies. I went so far as to get an interview at one of these encounter bars. Deep down in my heart, I wanted to prove to Daniel that I could make it in show business too. The man at the bar said I should get my husband's permission before I even thought of taking a job there. I suppose he didn't need irate spouses storming the place. To my surprise, Daniel didn't seem to mind the idea. Maybe it was the enormous amounts of money I could have earned that made the proposition even sweeter for him.

In the end I didn't have the nerve to take the job. I was really straight and insecure back then. I never felt pretty enough. So, instead of trying something different, I just kept taking secretarial jobs, which continued to make me feel degraded. Today, I'm not concerned about what anyone thinks of "Mistress Jacqueline" or about the profession I've chosen. The most degrading thing I've ever done didn't take place in a dungeon, but in countless office buildings, typing letters for asshole executives, dealing with hundreds of nasty customers from nine to five. I much prefer what I'm doing now, helping people to fulfill their sexual fantasies. Having a man worship my feet—and pay me quite generously for it—is much better than clerical work, let me tell you. At least I'm the one in control. I'm getting paid top money, and enjoying myself besides. In offices there are always idiots making you feel worthless just because you made a typo. Being a secretary was the most humiliating work on earth to me. I've never felt that for a moment being a Dominatrix.

In retrospect, if I had been daring enough to pursue exotic dancing and had felt better about my body (and myself), maybe my marriage with Daniel would have survived. At least both of us would have been working nights. But back then I was still consumed with the idea of being a "good girl" and a good wife. What does the good wife do? She goes along with whatever her husband says, grits her teeth, and makes believe everything is all right, even when it isn't.

Because I was so mixed up emotionally, I became an insomniac. I dreaded going to my job each morning so much that I couldn't sleep at night, sometimes for a week straight. I kept messing up even the most menial duties at my desk. I should have quit, but I was hung up on being responsible. I felt I had a responsibility to Daniel, but along the way, I'd forgotten about the responsibility I had to myself. After a string of sleepless nights, I was finally fired. My supervisor told me that she was doing me a favor. "I don't think you fit in here, Alice," she told me. Even though I understood what she meant, I was devastated. I didn't think I fit in anywhere. Sobbing, I broke down and called my mother. Thank God she was supportive, for once.

There was something about living with Daniel that punctured my self-esteem. In the beginning he had been very supportive, but that had changed. In the Virgin Islands, I had a lot of fun and felt good about myself, about my teaching skills. But the more I was with Daniel, and the deeper I fell in love with him, the less I concentrated on myself. His remarks about me being too heavy made me determined to lose weight. From pleasantly zaftig I dieted to a painfully thin eighty-eight pounds. I'd cook Daniel a hearty meat-and-potatoes dinner every night and sit across from him nibbling on a salad like a blonde gerbil. I knew it was driving Daniel crazy. It would have driven anyone crazy. There I was quickly making myself more imperfect instead of more perfect. I became a terrible bore, obsessively talking about losing pounds and inches. Everything I did, I did for Daniel. Around that time, we used to have this private joke—"Alice loves Daniel. And Daniel loves Daniel." I couldn't help but laugh. It was sad, but very true.

Being the responsible fool that I am, I began looking for another job immediately. Late one afternoon I found myself in front of the Industrial Finance building on California Street. On a whim I decided to visit the personnel department and explain my varied educational/secretarial background. The people in the office seemed very nice, and they were sure they had an interesting position right up my alley. With my teaching skills, they figured I'd do well in their training department. I was escorted upstairs to meet the head of the department, Carol. She was a real go-getter, a manly sort of woman. She explained that Mary Lou, the department coordinator, was getting ready to leave in a couple of months. Carol was looking for someone to step into Mary Lou's job after she left. It was an office environment, but at least I wouldn't be doing secretarial chores. At last, I'd be able to use my brain again.

As it turned out, I liked the work. The training department was a virtually new area and I was coordinating personnel and technical programs. It entailed a good deal of telephone work as I made hotel reservations for the people coming to town, set up the actual seminars, and made sure all of the proper equipment was available. I seemed to be good at this sort of detail-oriented work. I enjoyed seeing that everything flowed properly. There were even some freebies in it for me, like complimentary hotel suites.

Industrial Finance held great potential for my future. For a good year and a half, I was very happy. I knew that eventually I could be conducting classes on management and supervisory skills, the very thing I was now hiring people to do. In the meantime, I was teaching procedures on how to train people in loss-control techniques, casualty, and liability. Even though they sent me to some insurance classes, I really had no interest in this aspect of the business at all. I just couldn't seem to get behind it.

After a while, there were changes in the company that greatly affected my position. New people with more experience than I had were hired. I watched them climb past me in rank. Often, I had nothing to do except try to look busy. In my spare time I began to take acting classes and tennis lessons and work out at a local gym. There was Alice's life and there was Daniel's life. There was no connection between the two unless I tried to become a part of his.

At night, Daniel still frequented the comedy clubs. I'd accompany him whenever I could. After the initial excitement of his involvement, the scenario became pretty boring. To me, most of the other comedians seemed very clannish. I'm sure they thought I was a fifth wheel. I was seen as "The Wife." Although I didn't like playing that role, I didn't like sitting home alone at night either. When I had to get up early in the morning and rush to the office, Daniel would just sit around, read the paper, and linger over breakfast. That pissed me off! Eventually I became furious. I wanted Daniel to contribute to our lives financially. Lots of starving artists managed to have day jobs too. Occasionally, Daniel would get a job, but it would only last a few weeks. After a short trip to Mexico in which I footed the entire bill, Daniel felt guilty and promised adamantly that he'd start up his job hunt again. But he soon forgot his pledge. Looking back, I don't know why I didn't just pick up and leave him. Maybe I didn't think I had the right.

Although I tried my best to hide it, I was always angry. Anger is still a difficult emotion for me to express. Either I keep it inside or else I explode, but I've never learned to peacefully coexist with it. I finally looked up a therapist in the Yellow Pages. I needed someone to talk to, but the lady I chose was very cold and didn't seem to understand. I felt confined in her tiny office tucked away in the financial district. Before I stopped seeing her, she did tell me something that struck a sensitive chord. She pinpointed my desire to be everything for Daniel. "It's impossible," she said. "We can't possibly be everything for everybody. Sooner or later, he'll seek out someone else." It was a thought I couldn't deal with.

Daniel's friend Bobby came up with a scheme to go down to Los Angeles to audition for "The Gong Show." Of course, they went without me. Daniel happened to win and came back to San Francisco in full sail. "This is it! I'm on my way," he told me. Yes, but where, I wondered. Away from me? I was sure that if Daniel ever did become a successful comedian, he'd leave me. For that reason, I couldn't get enthusiastic about his future. It was something I was certain would sever us completely. For Daniel, the future seemed bright, but I was still a drudge. To this day I feel badly that I wasn't able to share Daniel's enthusiasm, but I was unhappy with my life, and had no real friends, no dreams of my own.

Down in L.A. Daniel had met a woman named Carol Haber. I hit the roof when she called him one night at midnight. Who was she? What had he done with her? Daniel admitted that he and Bobby had gone to a few dance clubs with her when they were in Los Angeles. Gone dancing! I loved to dance and Daniel always refused to take me. Besides occasional flare-ups like that, Daniel and I rarely fought. We were still friends, but it wasn't a growing, intimate relationship. Stagnant is a good word.

At least Daniel was beginning to get a few paying gigs. He met a guy named Ron Marks, who eventually became his writing partner. Ron is a big, fat, ugly, obnoxious, New-Yorker type. We didn't hit if off very well, but Daniel was drawn to him like a creative magnet, confident they were going to be the writing team of the eighties. Whatever small shred of encouragement they received was blown way out of proportion, proving they were the greatest thing since sliced bread. I'd have to sit around and listen to their incessant bragging. Drinking made this easier to bear.

Around that time Daniel became friendly with another writer, Doreen. Even though she had a good job with *San Francisco* magazine, Doreen had decided to move to L.A. This gave Daniel the bug to go also. I was really burned. I liked San Francisco and didn't want to leave. Everyone called L.A. "the Pits," full of phony people and smog. You were judged on the basis of how you looked, the kind of car you drove, and the people you knew. I didn't think I could deal with it. If I didn't want to go, Daniel made it clear that he would make the move without me.

Daniel should have never married me—or anyone. He was too immature, too selfish. But it was too late to think of that now. Although we rarely talked about breaking up, the subject would come up every now and then. I still couldn't believe he could just pick up and go without me. When Daniel became more insistent about the move, I started canvassing insurance companies in the area. Some responses were promising, especially an interview at Magic Mountain. The job entailed writing training programs on how to fix roller coasters. One of the perks was being able to go for rides during coffee breaks. One or two other companies expressed interest in hiring me, and then, all of a sudden, Daniel decided he didn't want to move after all. Living with Daniel was turning out to be an emotional roller-coaster ride in itself.

What could I do? Look for another job, of course. I found one at a company called "QWIK" a subsidiary of a major oil company. The company was going to produce a new line of word processors. Since I had a background in training, they were sure I'd be perfect to teach others how to design programs on how to train trainers. There was only one problem—I'm absolutely terrible with machines. Even though I had no computer background whatsoever, they convinced me not to worry about it. They wanted me to start "yesterday, if not sooner," so I immediately gave notice at Industrial and started at QWIK two weeks later.

Industrial had been a humane sort of company, but the folks at QWIK patterned themselves after IBM. The philosophy was steeped in hardcore sales. The offices were populated by an endless stream of men in blue striped suits. I didn't fit into that corporate mold at all. I tried my best to concern myself with my job, which was to teach, but first I had to learn how to use that damned machine. I sat in on training classes that didn't seem to do much good, so I convinced my boss to ship me east to an intense training program. Not only did I think it would be a nice little break, but I was sure I could swing a weekend trip to Manhattan. Or so I thought.

Giving the excuse that I was an insomniac, I avoided sharing a hotel room with a stranger, but dreams of goofing off were shattered when the instructor announced that this was a continuous, fourteen-day training program, complete with homework—no breaks, no weekends off. I managed to survive my incarceration by hanging out with the guys every night at the bar. I always managed to get shit-faced drunk. The day I had to make a presentation I was so hung over that I couldn't think straight. Needless to say, I was given one of the lowest grades in the history of the seminar. And no matter what I did I couldn't learn how to operate that infernal QWIK machine.

Back in San Francisco, my boss called me into his office. "What is it with you?" he asked. "I've gotten four calls about your behavior during the seminar. You're a troublemaker, aren't you?" He was smiling, but deadly serious. "Let's face it," he continued, "you just can't fit a square peg in a round hole." Since he'd convinced me to leave my last position, I was given two weeks' pay plus a glowing letter of recommendation. We shook hands and said goodbye.

That sudden change in our lives prompted Daniel to decide once again that we should move to Los Angeles. This time I was ready to go. Hoping to find a job in the *L.A. Times,* I came across an ad for a two-year work/study M.A. program in psychology at Pepperdine University. I made a deal with Daniel. If we went to L.A., I wanted to have the chance to finally do what I wanted to do. He agreed to work and help pay the bills while I took out a student loan to attend Pepperdine and worked part-time.

Luckily, Jenny and Will, friends of Bobby's parents, owned a beautiful home in Playa del Rey. They offered to let Daniel and I stay there until we found a place of our own. We lived in their lovely guest house and I jogged every day to the beach. Actually, it was a very nice beginning in a new place. In spite of myself, I liked Los Angeles.

I decided to do a bit of university shopping. I compared Pepperdine with Antioch University. To me, Antioch seemed to have a more laid-back, intellectual, free-thinking atmosphere. I knew it was my kind of place immediately. Everything seemed to be falling into place. Soon we moved into an apartment complex in Sherman Oaks, right in the San Fernando Valley. Life with Daniel seemed very happy for a while.

Los Angeles was very "real" about show business. San Francisco seemed to be populated by a bunch of kids trying to make jokes and being very uppity about it. In L.A., being funny was a very profitable business. The evidence was in the black Mercedes cars that choked the streets, the shops on Rodeo Drive. A friend of Daniel's introduced him to a man named Jackie. An old-time comedian, he used to open up Elvis Presley's show. Jackie now managed comedy writers and was very good at it. Since that's where Daniel's real talents lie, Jackie agreed to manage the writing team of Daniel and Ron Marks, who was now officially Daniel's writing partner. When Daniel took me to see Jackie in his office, I finally felt included. I wasn't just a silly wife on the sidelines, but a vital part of the union. Jackie didn't make me wait outside. He recognized me as Daniel's wife. Jackie himself had been married for many years. For the first time, I thought there might be some kind of stability in the comedy business. Not just waiting around, bullshitting, doing gigs, running here, running there, and thinking, "I'm great!" In L.A., comedy was an industry. People had families. I was suddenly feeling much better about Daniel's career choice.

Ironically, the first thing Jackie did was secure Daniel a comedy gig back in San Francisco. I was pleased because I assumed I'd be able to go up north with him for a visit, too. I hadn't yet started school and had nothing much to do. But Daniel became very wild-eyed at the suggestion of me accompanying him. "You only care about yourself," he screamed. Grabbing me, he slammed my face against the wall. I collapsed to the floor, sobbing. Daniel started sobbing that he was sorry, crying and apologizing. I blamed myself for provoking him and insisted that I was sorry, too. We were both very confused, but it was me who had the bruises and a very sore black eye.

Ron arrived a few minutes later. Pulling Daniel aside, he suggested that we needed psychiatric help. I didn't think our situation was that serious, though, and tried to convince myself that Daniel would never hurt me again. Actually, it was the only episode of physical violence we ever experienced. "If you knew how much I really loved you," Daniel kept saying over and over again. But if he cherished me, then why did he always manage to make me feel like shit? I explained that all I really wanted was for him to include me in his life a little bit more. Make me feel like an important, integral part. It didn't seem too difficult.

Instead, Daniel made me feel even more insecure. Whenever we went out together, he would blatantly stare at other women. Once, on the ballfield, a woman came up and started flirting with Daniel right in front of me. She knew damned well that I was his wife. If the situation were reversed, no man would ever dare do that in front of a woman's husband. Men seem to respect spousal situations a lot more than women do. After I was married, single guys seemed to ignore me, especially if Daniel was around, as though my wedding band set off electric shocks in their testicles. But for some reason, women act differently, as though married guys are prey, a real challenge to capture. It's not a matter of possession. It's a matter of respect.

After I started attending school I felt much better about myself. I was involved in something other than Daniel. I felt worthy again. But at the very start of classes at Antioch, I did feel uncomfortable. Everyone seemed so intelligent, so much smarter than me. Even though I probably knew as much as any other student, I felt inferior. Classes were very small and we were encouraged to vent our opinions. We were also expected to write emotion-oriented papers. Another requirement was that all candidates for a masters in psychology had to be in therapy. The school had a real "know thyself" policy. Antioch was a more intense, intimate school than Boston University. I made a few close, deep friendships with fellow students.

During the fourth year of our marriage, for the first time, Daniel became less important to me. I finally had a grip on myself, a focus. I read diligently, did my homework, went to field-study internships. Because I was so immersed in my studies, in some way our marriage became better. But I also realized that in pursuing vastly different careers, Daniel and I were growing further apart. My eyes and my emotions were opened. I found myself suddenly conscious of the other guys in my classes. Handsome faces. Tempting bodies. Alluring minds. There was one man in particular, Karl. I rediscovered the fun of having a harmless crush, the silly, breathless, fluttery feeling that comes with it. I felt like a woman again. Karl and I became good friends, nothing more. Karl was basically a happy-go-lucky type, not the least bit interested in getting seriously involved with me. But it was fun to look at him and daydream.

Suddenly I was developing a real social life again. I'd often accompany classmates to bars or go dancing with them. Any relationship becomes strained when one person starts to grow and the other stays the same. My therapist told me that I probably had some underlying feelings of anger toward Daniel. Of course I did! Besides that, our sex life had almost ceased. Daniel never took the initiative, and even when I made innuendoes, Daniel would brush me off. Oh, we'd still hug and kiss and talk to each other. But most of the time during the last year of our marriage I felt as though I was Daniel's buddy, not his wife. I definitely wasn't feeling sexual toward Daniel anymore, but I couldn't figure out what was wrong. Whenever I tried to discuss it with him, he insisted things between us were fine. I couldn't understand why I was the only one in the relationship who felt that way. When I'd ask him why we weren't having sex, he'd say because he was tired or something like that.

After we moved to Los Angeles, our sex life really started going downhill. Before that, we enjoyed what you might call basic, traditional sex. We even rated our fucks, good session or bad session. But something was always lacking for me. Although Daniel was very proficient at making me climax with his hands, he would never kiss or lap my pussy. Oral sex was something I really liked, but Daniel didn't. He'd use his hands, diddling my clit, but I often had the feeling that he was just doing it to appease me, silently wondering, "When the hell is she going to cum?" with his wrist aching. I always had an orgasm, eventually. Something was lacking, though. I wasn't sure what. But Daniel still maintained the facade of marriage. I was eager to discuss our problems after a therapy session, but he'd always assure me that everything was fine. Better than ever. Understandably, that always made me crazy. Everything wasn't fine!

Toward the end of my graduate school, Daniel had some work in New York. After months of having no sex with my husband and having the hots for Karl, I was determined to have a wild fling. Karl lived in Malibu and was asking me to come out to visit. I kept making up all kinds of excuses, but finally relented—the day before Daniel came home. Driving through the Canyon, I suddenly felt alive again. I felt sexual again. I was free! But, of course, I'd picked the worst time. Karl was a guitarist and he was getting ready to leave for a club date. What a disappointment. I had decided that I was going to fuck him and didn't want to leave until I got my wish, so I sat through two hours of his music in a ratty little bar. When Karl and I finally crawled into bed, it was almost over before it began. I was aching to really make slow, languid love, to taste his body, to kiss for a long time. But Karl was incredibly aroused. His hands grazed my breasts and belly, a quick prerequisite to climbing on top of me and getting inside. I didn't climax, not even close. Although it was something of a letdown after desiring Karl for so long, I was elated that I'd finally done something forbidden that I really wanted to do.

Not being in a corporate environment where drinking is acceptable, even expected, my alcohol consumption tapered off. After classes, a bunch of us would go out, but it was usually for tea or coffee so we could passionately discuss the complexities of our psyches. I honestly didn't miss drinking, but I still had to rely on a glass of wine to lull me to sleep. Karl was trying to use biofeedback to help me cut down. For a while I actually stopped drinking altogether, but it didn't last very long.

My time at Antioch was a happy one. Life was normal. Although I was still a bit bothered by my spanking fantasies, I tried to deal with them. They weren't going to disappear. Many times when Daniel and I were making love, I'd envision him spanking me. One night I summoned up a heap of courage and asked if he'd do it. I could tell by the look on his face that he thought it was enormously silly, but he went along with it. He really didn't understand it. Daniel laid me flat on my belly, took a hairbrush, and began whacking my ass really hard—too hard. It hurt and there was nothing erotic about it. I was screaming. After a few whacks, he stopped. In a disgusted voice, he said, "Forget it." Maybe he had some fantasies of his own that he couldn't deal with. Maybe some fantasies are better left unspoken.

Once, in his tiny Village apartment, Daniel had grabbed me suddenly as he sat on the toilet lid, put me over his knee and spanked me playfully. I didn't have the nerve to let him know how much I loved it. Then there had been an episode before we left San Francisco. Although Daniel rarely indulged in drugs, one afternoon we each took a Quaalude. Those pills are famous for making people very aroused. Walking through Golden Gate Park hand in hand, Daniel admitted that he liked the sensation of being high and horny. Because we were both feeling very passionate I was able to tell him, "Spank me. Now. Please!" Daniel was only too happy to drag me to the bushes and fuck me, but he wouldn't spank me. Still wandering through the park, Daniel ran into his baseball buddies. I was mortified when he started yelling to them, "Guess what my wife wanted me to do? Spank her!" I could have died right there. My husband and his friends were laughing at my most clandestine passion.

When I finally told my therapist about my mild S&M fantasies, I could barely choke out the words. My face was gleaming red. I could feel it. Starting to sweat, I held onto my hands and stammered, "I enjoy being spanked," as though it were the most heinous sin in the universe. At first, he didn't know what to say. Then, very grimly, he explained that when my self-esteem grew, I'd lose the desire to be punished. End of story. I realize now that he really didn't understand the concept of submission and dominance. The very thought probably terrified him. Like Freud, I'm sure he labeled that type of behavior perverse and deviant.

My therapist's reaction to my deepest, darkest secret made me feel many things, most prominently anger. He knew everything about me, perhaps more than even Daniel did. How dare he sit there and judge me by one tiny facet of my personality? I began to realize there was a need for someone who understands the delicate intricacies of S&M fantasies. I was sure I could get people who were immersed in S&M to talk about their emotions. I would never be embarrassed by someone's admission, as my therapist had been. I knew how devastating that could be. There is a validity in all of our sexual desires—in the man who wants to worship feet, in the woman who craves being whipped, in the man who wants to dress up like a woman and crawl into a female's sensibilities. Nothing is wrong or bad or ugly between consenting adults. I honestly don't think anything would mortify me. In fact, I applaud the courage in people who say, "I'm different. But love me, accept me anyway. Please." I am one of those people.

6

Abandonment

I was class valedictorian when I graduated from Antioch, and really pleased to be rewarded with the honor of speaking at the graduation ceremonies. Ironically, it fell on the day of my fifth wedding anniversary. Daniel was in the audience. Afterward, we went to our favorite restaurant. It had all the makings of a memorable day, but I felt a great deal of emptiness inside. There were a lot of empty feelings that year. I had tried to cover them up with a quick affair the previous March. I ended up fucking one of my fellow graduate students in his car after a party. In a school with such a relaxed atmosphere, making love came quite naturally.

Educationally speaking, I wasn't satisfied with just having a masters degree. Anxious and determined to get my doctorate, I was disappointed that Antioch didn't have a Ph.D. program. The other schools I visited were a little too mainstream for my taste. I had plans to continue my studies, but put them on hold for a while.

I put them on hold for almost eight years, as it turned out. I have finally started studying for my Ph.D. at the Institute for the Advanced Study of Human Sexuality in San Francisco. I love the feeling of both physical and mental intimacy in the classes. It reminds me of *The Harrad Experiment,* not just the sex, but the fact that there is so much communication, so much connection between people, not only in bed, but everywhere. I distinctly remember a scene in the book when one of the guys was inside Beth Hillyer. They were physically joined, but were in no hurry to climax, very pleased with verbally communicating while they made love, laughing, with lots of emotion. This scene stimulated me mentally. That's the way I think sex should be, something shared between friends, between people who care about each other —not just "getting off," or with "scoring." Sex isn't a game of rivalry. You don't score points. There should be a feeling of true intimacy, closeness, and communication. That is what I've always wanted and sought, but rarely achieved. The institute has that kind of atmosphere. Even if a Ph.D. doesn't add up to me actually becoming a psychotherapist, I'm sure that just the experience of being at the institute will mean a lot to me personally.

But all that is later. During what would turn out to be the last few months of my marriage to Daniel, the Writers' Guild went on strike. Daniel and Ron finally went their separate ways. Daniel was spending more and more time with Doreen, the writer he'd known in San Francisco. Like us, she had relocated to L.A. I liked Doreen. At the time, she was living with an actor named Daryl Anderson. You might remember him as "Animal," the photographer on the old "Lou Grant" television show. Although Doreen held down a secretarial job, she had an idea for a screenplay that she and Daniel began fleshing out immediately. In a short time, they became inseparable.

I thought nothing of it. Even though Daniel and I weren't making love very often, he was very loving toward me. I never felt threatened by Daniel and Doreen's relationship. My major criterion in those days as far as jealousy went was how thin someone was. Because Doreen was heavier than me, I quickly dismissed her as being no competition. But I did realize that she and Daniel had much in common. "What are we doing together?" I'd often ask Daniel, half joking, half not. "It should be you and Doreen." But Daniel told me all of the nice things he told Doreen about me. He kept telling me how much he loved me. I didn't realize it, but I suppose Doreen and Daniel were lovers even then.

Although they usually worked at Doreen's boy friend's place, I came home one day to find them in our apartment. The way they both looked at me made me feel like a stranger in my own apartment, as though I were intruding. There was a definite "we" feeling that I was not a part of. They made it very clear. I tried to immerse myself in my own career. It started with another frantic search for a job. I left nothing unconsidered, including things like being a nutrition counselor. At least

I would be counseling *something*. Soon I was accepted in an intern program that promised to help me build up a private practice as a psychologist. In addition, I began to organize workshops with my friend Kerry from graduate school. Specializing in women's groups, we'd speak on all the current issues: How to build self-esteem, overcoming shyness, and dressing for success were among the most popular. I was very busy and involved, almost too busy to worry about Daniel and Doreen.

In the beginning of August, my sister Robin and her husband Bob came out to visit for a few days. They arrived on a Saturday, and I'd planned to spend that night entertaining them. But Daniel had other plans. He'd bought tickets to see the movie *Napoleon,* not to take me, but to take Doreen. So Daniel and I went our separate ways for the evening. I took Robin and Bob on a typical L.A. night on the town— dinner and the Improv comedy club. During the past months, I had grown used to socializing without Daniel, so it didn't bother me in the least.

Sunday, Robin and Bob were celebrating their wedding anniversary and Daniel promised to spend the occasion with all of us. The day progressed much like any other. Jane Fonda's workout centers had just come to the Valley and I'd become an avid member. As usual, I woke up early to attend the nine a.m. class. An adorable instructor named Ed was more of an incentive than the idea of staying in shape. Talking to him afterward about his recent breakup with his girlfriend, I arrived home later than I usually did. Daniel was still lying in bed, poring over the Sunday paper, when I walked into the apartment. I kissed him hello, ate my breakfast, and made a quick stop in the bathroom. Then I crawled into bed to cuddle with him just as I always did. I was fondling Daniel's cock when he pulled away.

"What's wrong?" I asked, following him across the room.

"Nothing," he insisted.

Daniel's face was ashen. I couldn't imagine what was troubling him. When I asked him again, he said, "I think you'd better sit down." Obediently, I plopped down on the edge of the bed. Daniel took a deep breath.

"I called my brother Harry yesterday," he explained. "I told him that I'm leaving you."

My mouth must have fallen open in shock. I couldn't find words at first. A veil of tears was blurring my eyes, clogging my throat.

"What?" I asked in disbelief.

"I'm leaving you," Daniel repeated coldly.

I didn't know what to say. Like a fool, I heard myself apologizing. "I'm sorry, Daniel. I'm so sorry. I must have done something wrong. I must have done something to make you want to leave me. Whatever it was, I'm sorry."

I was babbling like an idiot. I can't even recall half of what I said. "I'm sorry," I muttered. "So sorry for whatever I did."

Still, he was unmoved. "No," he said.

It was so pitiful. So sad. "Please don't leave me," I begged. "Please don't leave me here alone. I don't know what I'd do without you."

But Daniel wouldn't even hold me. Was it too sickening to even touch me anymore? "No. You don't understand," he said. "It's not that simple. I have to. That's all."

"Is there someone else involved, Daniel?"

"It doesn't matter," he told me and walked out of the bedroom.

Half blind with tears, I dragged myself to my feet and followed him. Daniel was sitting grimly on the living room floor. I sat down beside him.

"Who is it?" I asked, trembling. Suddenly, I saw everything very clearly. I answered my own question. "It's Doreen, isn't it?"

"She's leaving Daryl," Daniel said, so coolly. "We're planning to live together."

I was confused. "But how are you going to support the both of us?" I wondered aloud. Like a child.

"I'm not," Daniel said simply. "Look, Alice. Remember how you keep telling me that you miss the way it used to be, the times when we couldn't get enough of each other? Well, that's the way it is now with me and Doreen. We can't get enough of each other."

My heart just dropped. The ache between my ribs was almost unbearable. I felt as though I were living in the midst of the worst nightmare imaginable, only I couldn't wake up. No matter what I did, I couldn't wake up. Somewhere in the distance, I heard Daniel's voice again. "You can have all the furniture. I'll take my things out as soon as possible." My things. His things. How could I sleep in our bed alone?

Daniel was insane enough to suggest that we go out with Robin and my brother-in-law that night, just as planned. We didn't have to tell them anything, not yet. Create an illusion. Act out a happy little scenario. But he had already made up his mind to go. Nothing could make him change it. Once again, Daniel had made a huge decision without me. I just wanted to know how long he and Doreen had been together. How long had I been so stupid? "We've only been lovers for two weeks," Daniel told me. I'm still not sure whether I believe him or not. "But it's love, Alice. We're certain of that."

To this day I cringe whenever I think about that morning. Even though Daniel and I had problems and were growing apart, I still *liked* Daniel. He was my best friend, my sometimes lover, my confidant. He knew me inside out. I felt betrayed.

Even with all of those negative emotions coursing through my body, I realized that I had an intense desire for Daniel sexually. It was overpowering. Suddenly, I wanted him to make love to me. I needed to have him inside me. "Please fuck me, Daniel," I begged hoarsely.

"I can't," he said. "I love Doreen."

I was weeping again. "Then get the hell out of here!" I screamed. "I don't care where the hell you go. Just get out!"

Crying hysterically, I somehow made it over to Robin's hotel room. I have no recollection of driving there, only of falling into my sister's arms when she opened the door. I didn't know what to think or feel. My values, my life, were crumbling around me like sand.

Bob drove to our apartment to have a talk with Daniel. They didn't argue or fight. Daniel just calmly talked as he packed his things. He'd made a decision. No one could sway him. "Maybe if we'd had kids, this never would have happened," he said. Had a family? Whenever I told Daniel that I wanted a child, it was quickly dismissed because he never had a steady job. Then there was the all-important comedy career he was trying to pursue. That always came first.

The hours passed. I felt as though I were under water, watching everything swirl around me and listening to my brother-in-law talk. "Don't worry," Bob promised, "Daniel will get tired of Doreen. He'll come crawling back to you by Rosh Hashana."

But Daniel never came back. To blot up my brain, I drank Amaretto until four in the morning. Robin tried to convince me to munch on something while they had dinner, but how could I eat? I wanted to die. If I couldn't die, then I didn't want to feel anything. I wanted to drink until my heart was numb. When I was sufficiently wasted, of course, my car decided not to budge. I had to wait around for a jump start from AAA. Coming home to an empty apartment was the oddest feeling. I dreaded going to bed alone, so I took a Valium to help me relax. Maybe I wouldn't wake up the next morning. I did, but taking that pill was equivalent to jumping off a cliff. It was the start of much craziness. That's when the real insanity began.

I felt lost. Talking to Doreen's abandoned boyfriend, Daryl, offered some consolation. But he understood only a fraction of what I was feeling. He described how Doreen had packed her things and met Daniel at our place. Daryl was almost as shocked to learn about their affair as I had been. He and Doreen were planning to get married, going so far as to buy a home in North Hollywood. Sometimes things change fast.

I couldn't seem to eat. The only thing I could hold down was carob chips. Buying them by the bagful from the health food store, I'd munch on them as soon as I woke up. I'd munch on them as I spoke on the telephone all morning. I especially liked talking to Audrey. She was also a therapist and had been divorced for a few years. Her area of expertise was physically abused women. We would sit there and joke that there should be something called "Wedding Album Therapy." Even at the shelter for abused women battered victims would often show up with no possessions other than their wedding albums. Their husbands could have broken their noses, smashed their ribs, it didn't matter. They liked to look at the pretty pictures in the albums. Audrey and I laughed, but we had to admit that in the quiet of our empty apartments, we often did the same thing. Fools. My other friends tried to be understanding, but I could barely function. The only activity I could manage was working out. I did aerobics morning, noon, and night, sometimes taking three or four classes a day. That way I didn't have to think. I pushed my body relentlessly.

For some reason, I phoned Daniel's parents even before I spoke to my own. Frankly, I didn't think my folks would care very much. I thought they'd probably rattle on about how they never liked Daniel anyway. Daniel's parents were angry with him. They didn't know what to say or how to console me. I knew I would miss them. No matter how they felt, Daniel was still their son. I kept putting off speaking to my own parents. Finally, I asked Robin to phone them and explain everything. To my surprise, they called me immediately and were very understanding. Just as I'd thought, Mom stressed how they had never really liked Daniel. "Should we come out there to be with you?" my mother asked, somewhat halfheartedly. If they really cared, they would have been on a plane immediately. They knew I was all alone. But I told them I was all right.

I was very confused. Part of me was excited about the breakup. I hadn't had the courage to leave Daniel, but now I was free. Dutifully attending my exercise class the day after Daniel left, I was almost looking forward to telling the instructor, Frank, about my plight. When I began to cry, he wrapped his arms around me. In spite of myself, I felt aroused. Part of me wanted to be comforted. Another part wanted to be fucked into oblivion.

The next day, I was determined to seduce Frank. After his seven o'clock class, I practically out and out propositioned him. Frank was very sweet. He kissed me on the forehead. "I find you very attractive, Alice," he explained. "But it's too soon. I don't want to be revenge on your husband." Frank left me there, standing in the parking lot. I guess he was right. I wouldn't be happy if the situation were reversed. But what the hell was I going to do with myself?

7

Abandon

I had discovered a decadent thrill a few months earlier. As part of an assignment for a human sexuality class at Antioch, we were instructed to explore something different sexually, something we'd never done before. It could be as mainstream as going to a pornographic movie or as offbeat as visiting a transvestite club. I decided to take a peek at a strip joint in the Valley called the "Queen Mary." Although they specialized in transvestite shows Wednesdays through Sundays, I attended on a Tuesday—male stripper night.

The noisy room was teeming with both men and women. The atmosphere was totally loose. A man named Ronnie was the first on stage. Dancing to "Great Balls of Fire" and "Splish Splash," he actually climbed into a bathtub on stage. He had sandy hair, warm, romantic eyes, and a delicately sinewy build. I thoroughly enjoyed watching Ronnie gyrate. After a few drinks, I was brave enough to wave a dollar bill just like many of the other women were. To my surprise, Ronnie sauntered over and thrust his pelvis at me. Graspng my head in his hands, he rewarded me with a passionate, open-mouthed kiss as I tucked the money into his scant briefs. After that I was hooked on the Queen Mary. The phenomenon of women watching men strip at these clubs intrigued me enough to make it the focus of a paper for my sexuality class. Of course, this revolved around my own desires.

Sam was one dancer I particularly enjoyed. Muscular, with red hair, he billed himself as the "Exotic Psychotic." As a budding psychologist,

I was sure I could cure his ills, and then some. Sam came on stage wearing a straitjacket, hung himself from a hook on a rafter and proceeded to wiggle and squirm his way out of his confines. (Was it light bondage?) But it wasn't his act that turned me on incredibly—it was his body. Sam was much more of a tease than the others, plus he had a cocky attitude I found myself drawn to.

At the end of the night the performers would all dance on a ledge above the bar. Customers were encouraged to get up and give them one last tip. I looked at Sam longingly, but didn't dare do more. Suddenly he summoned me silently with a curve of his index finger, a subtle act of dominance that hooked me. I went to him immediately.

There wasn't much small talk."What are you doing after the show?" Sam asked bluntly.

I told him I had just broken up with my husband. Sam had recently left his girlfriend, Marcy. It seemed perfect. "Do you want me to come home with you?" he wondered.

I was in a state of wonderful anticipation and cold terror as I waited for Sam to get dressed. He followed my car on his motorcycle as we wound through the roads in the Valley. It was like a fantasy. At one point Sam motioned for me to roll down the window. He shouted into the wind. "By the way, do you like to have your pussy eaten?" The shock of those words gave me an even warmer oozing between my thighs. Oral sex was something I loved—something Daniel would never do.

We had incredible sex that night. Sam really knew how to make love to a woman. One of the most aggressive and yet sensual lovers I'd ever experienced, he also liked to talk and encouraged me to let him know what I wanted. After seven years making love to a man who lacked imagination, sex had become a rote act. This was miraculous. Instead of refusing to bury his head between my thighs, Sam seemed to savor it. Unlike an encounter with Daniel, sex wasn't over in twenty minutes. It was two hours of Sam bringing me to incredible peaks and then gently setting me down.

Halfway through the night, a horrible thought occurred to me. What if this was all too good to be true? What if Sam was expecting to get paid? Somehow, I dared to come right out and ask. Sam just looked at me and laughed. "I'd be a pretty bad whore if I didn't ask for my money up front, wouldn't I?"

That night with Sam certainly boosted my drooping self-esteem.

I knew we weren't about to embark on a "relationship," but I was grateful to discover that I could respond completely to a man. Sam tried to be sweet about what had happened with Daniel, understanding how much it must have crushed me. He noticed that I had virtually stopped eating. Very romantically, Sam fed me fruits and took care of me for a short time.

Daniel and I had no real contact. I went ahead and changed the locks on the doors. I suppose that's the first thing you do when someone leaves. The only time he phoned was to get some of his possessions. His baseball cleats. He even had the nerve to take some meat he'd bought. I wanted Daniel out of my life and wasn't about to keep letting him burst in whenever he wanted. Daniel never had kind words, even when he called for permission to stop by. And there was always Doreen's voice in the background, priming him, telling him what to say.

Although I had my new degree and was diligently searching for a job, a part of me had no idea what I was doing. I was going crazy thinking about Daniel, desiring Sam's caress, and hating Daniel all at once. I had once hoped that at this point I would be able to fall back on Daniel's career while I built up a private practice. But with Daniel gone, seeking a Ph.D. was out of the question for the time being. My parents began sending me money. I didn't want to accept it, but I had no choice. All in all, it was a very confusing time emotionally.

My first Sunday as a single woman I went to the marina with Kerry and her divorced mother. It was a typical singles stakeout. It was almost as though I had awakened from a dream. Suddenly I was aware of all the single women that surrounded me. There seemed to be an entire tribe of us cramming the restaurant in war paint in the form of mascara and lipstick, stalking, hoping. Would I be alone for the rest of my life? From that moment on, I became a carefree party girl. During the day I struggled to build up a private practice as a therapist. At night I did whatever felt good. I went to Jane Fonda's at least twice a day. Getting much-needed emotional support from my classmates, I was also the thinnest and tightest I'd ever been. Oh, I might have been torn apart on the inside, but on the outside, I looked great! It didn't take long for me to bounce back, as usual. After every trauma in my life, I have never given myself a chance to squirm in my sorrow. Maybe that's how I survive. Either I'm very stupid or very strong. I'm not sure which.

Finding Sam helped, but it didn't last long. Our fucking was certainly hot, but there was nothing else. Once we even planned a regular Saturday night date. I dashed out to buy a new outfit for the occasion. We agreed to meet in a coffee shop near where Sam lived. I arrived all dressed up and looking cute. He hadn't arrived yet. I waited. And I waited. I called him at home repeatedly, but kept getting his answering machine. This went on for an hour. Meanwhile I had to brush off an obnoxious man who insisted on trying to pick me up. Sitting there alone, sipping tepid coffee, I finally told the waitress my plight. She looked at me knowingly. "Welcome to single life in L.A.," she said.

Sam never did show up. The next day there was a flimsy excuse in the guise of a wild story, some crazy saga about a friend getting robbed, blah, blah. That was the end of Sam, but I kept visiting the Qween Mary. There were plenty of other dancers to choose from. That became my personal challenge, my quest, going to the club night after night seeing how many dancers I could collect.

Next was Steven. On stage he billed himself as "Heavin' Steven." He came out dressed like a hardhat. He'd take a tape measure out of his pants and you'd watch it grow and grow, wondering if his cock was doing the same. Before my fling with Sam I had concluded that these men were probably uneventful in bed. Since they'd probably burned out most of the sexual energy on stage, there might not be much left afterward. But, happily, I discovered that this wasn't true. Steven was just as good a fuck as Sam.

My drinking and drug use escalated tremendously. I'm certain that's what allowed me to be so free with my body without so much as an afterthought. That's exactly what happened with a guy a female instructor at Jane Fonda's set me up with. I drove over to his place and guzzled a few drinks. The next thing I knew we were screwing on his floor and I was half wondering how I'd gotten there. These men were just one-nighters. No one took me seriously. No one imagined that there was a hurt little girl hiding behind the mask of a carefree slut. They wanted me. I gave them what they wanted. All the while I thought I was having fun. I was a therapist, but I was in dire need of one myself. My brain was boggled. And in spite of myself I was still very much in love with Daniel.

But love or not, I knew I had to get an attorney. I didn't really need one, but I was so angry at Daniel that I wanted to get back at him. I wanted to make the divorce as difficult as possible for him. I wanted to make him hurt as much as I was hurting. Pretty soon, our lawyers were arguing back and forth. One of their biggest brawls was over an ancient hi-fi set. It was clearly Daniel's (a gift from his father when Daniel was a teenager), but I pretended that I wanted it. All of my fury, all of my feelings of betrayal were focused on the battle for that stupid little record player. Never once did Daniel and I ever sit down and discuss the disintegration of our marriage. The only time we came close was when we were forced to file our income taxes together that year. Meeting him to sign papers, I made sure I looked as attractive as I could. Daniel was cold, pretending not to notice. Reluctantly, he agreed to have a cup of coffee with me. "I left because you put me on a pedestal, Alice. You made me into something that I just couldn't be," he tried to explain. "I was too much a part of your life." These things were surely true in the beginning of our marriage, but not when it began to fall apart. Why didn't he just *tell me before it was too late*? Maybe I could have changed. Maybe we could have worked on it. I think the real problem was that in the final months of our relationship I *wasn't* putting Daniel on a pedestal. He missed that. I was changing, and he couldn't deal with my independence.

Months later Daniel stopped by to drop off some sort of paperwork. I arranged for a girlfriend to be there too because I didn't want to be alone with him. My rage toward Daniel wasn't so intense anymore. Perhaps I'd softened, but I finally allowed Daniel to take his beloved hi-fi. Daniel just looked at me very sadly. "Oh, Boobie . . ." he said, and his voice trailed off. That was one of his silly pet names for me. I couldn't bear to hear it again and burst out crying. Daniel and I silently held each other for a few moments. Then he was gone.

The terrible sadness of the situation continued to plague me—the unresolved things, the unsaid words. It's difficult for me to understand how Daniel could have loved me and yet have simply walked out of my life. I still wish Daniel and I could be friends. I'd love to be able to phone him and chat about our lives, just to know how he's doing. Maybe I should feel more angry toward him than I do, but I've never felt very comfortable expressing anger. About a week after Daniel left, I tried to confront my feelings in an encounter group. It was a wonderful Saturday afternoon class headed by Lou Yablonsky. His technique was something called psychodrama, a very intense form of therapy where people dramatically reenact traumatic pieces of their lives.

Another person acts as your alter-ego and says the things you might be thinking, but dare not even speak. Other people assume the roles of the antagonists and you confront them as you were never able to in the actual situation.

Lou began by talking about relationships in general. I had hidden myself way in the back of the classroom. Suddenly I felt Lou's eyes burning right through me. "Why do I feel as though I'm talking directly to you?" Lou asked. With a deep breath, I explained that my husband had walked out on me the week before. I was the perfect candidate to enact the first psychodrama.

Two people in the group played the part of Daniel. One man played Early Daniel, the Daniel during our happy days in New York. Another played Late Daniel, the cruel, brooding man I'd been married to all those years. One girl even played Doreen. We were encouraged to use a "bataka"—a foam-rubber pillow—to express our anger. In this controlled setting, we could lash out, hit, hurt, and scream, if we wanted to. Even though I was sobbing, even though I was furious, I had a lot of trouble expressing any sort of anger toward the Doreen character. I hit her once or twice, halfheartedly. But that was all. I couldn't even direct symbolic cruelty at my enemies.

After Daniel and I split up the major thing I focused my energies upon was getting my marriage/family/child counselor license. In the state of California, before you can practice, you must have a masters degree in clinical psychology, which I had just gotten. Then you need three thousand hours of clinical experience. Finally, you have to pass written and oral exams. While I was still at Antioch I participated in two internship programs that added up to a few hours, but I needed many more.

I became a paraprofessional counselor at the Southern California Counseling Center. Supervised by trained professionals, I had a regular client load. Just as I'd surmised, I really enjoyed being a therapist. I discovered that I had a lot of compassion for people and also that I possessed good listening skills. But the base salary made it difficult for me to make a decent living. I knew I needed an additional income, but the search for another job was fruitless. Hospitals tended to hire people with masters degrees in social work, not clinical psychology. As a result, I floundered about in a multitude of unsatisfactory part-time jobs. One was in a school for emotionally disturbed children, a scary place to work because the kids were often rough. Since I'm tiny, it wasn't easy to subdue the students physically. Then there was a program for schizophrenics. The idea was to keep them in a home environment supervised by a team that monitored them from morning to night. Because we were trying to mainstream them into society, they also had to hold down a job. I had two patients in my charge. One had to be escorted to his car-washing job daily. The only problem was that *I'd* end up doing the washing while he sat in my car, hearing strange sounds and voices that kept calling out to him. Another guy wasn't schizophrenic, but chronically depressed. It was no wonder, because he was tremendously obese. His escape mechanism was eating himself to distraction. His job was landscaping at a local Shakey's Pizza Parlor. All day I'd have to sit and watch this huge man bending over, tending to the lawn. Understandably, I found this type of work incredibly stifling. I had my masters but was breaking my back in a hodgepodge of jobs that paid only seven or eight dollars an hour.

One day I got a promising offer that would both help me build up a practice and teach me how to organize workshops. A man named Fred Schafter called me. Only twenty-nine, he was a graduate of Antioch and in the process of looking for a "very special intern" to share his practice. He invited both Kerry and me to come down for an interview. During our meeting I became certain that Fred was not only impressed with my credentials but also attracted to me as a woman. Kerry didn't like him at all, immediately pegging him as a pushy shyster. I found Fred very handsome, and intriguing as well. I was also impressed by his cool manner and his posh Santa Monica offices. That same evening Fred phoned me and offered me the job. He promised that he could help me build up a practice and would steer much of his client base in my direction. He was already enormously successful giving classes in self-hypnosis. As a bonus, he would teach the craft to me so I could also cash in on the phenomenon. It was the most exciting offer I'd had in a long time.

Working with Fred turned out to be a huge mistake. He talked a good game, but wound up doing absolutely nothing for me. A lot of things were left unsaid in the beginning. I soon discovered that I had to pay for his supposed skill and knowledge. As an intern, I was required to have a supervisor. Fred agreed to be mine, but I had to pay him forty dollars a week for the privilege, and also had to pay him rent for office space when I saw clients. It wasn't really a partnership at all. There were no referrals. Like a used-car salesman of the psychology world, Fred was constantly marketing himself. Everywhere we went, he handed people his brochure. He even persuaded me to go to local shopping malls to give them out. I was a lost soul in search of a mentor. Fred gladly filled that slot. The sexual chemistry between us continued to smolder, but I knew he wasn't available. Everyone knew that. Fred was living with Sally, one of the most brilliant teachers at Antioch. She was at least twelve years older than him.

But Fred's involvement with Sally didn't stop us from getting involved. For two weeks we stared longingly at each other, our mutual desire silently boiling below the surface. Fred's deep blue eyes penetrated me to the core. By the end of the two weeks we were lovers. "What are we going to do about this mad chemistry between us?" he asked bluntly one day. By that night, we were fucking away on top of his desk.

It was a hot, fleshy relationship. We'd stay at the office until three or four in the morning. On my knees, I'd take him in my mouth as he sat behind his messy desk. Or he'd fling my skirt up over my hips and take me from behind, right there on the carpet. Afterwards, we'd both go home to our separate residences. I didn't mind sharing Fred at first, especially after the mess with Daniel. In a way, it was a safe relationship for me, because I knew Fred was already involved with Sally. I didn't have to worry about him chasing another woman, because I *was* the other woman. In the circumstances, I liked that role better.

I fell head over heels for Fred, even though he still made me pay him for the privilege of being my supervisor. I admired him, wanted to be like him, and wanted to learn from him. But Fred turned out to be one more guy who made me feel that nothing I ever did was good enough. Often, when I spoke to a client over the telephone, Fred would pull me aside later and tell me how I could improve my phone manner. Then he'd turn around and tell me what great potential I had. He continually spouted confusing, mixed messages. Fred's practice was flourishing. His appointment book was always filled, but he never funneled any clients in my direction, as he'd promised.

To complicate matters, Sally found out about our affair. I suppose we weren't doing much to hide it. Everyone around us knew and it was only a matter of time before Sally found out. I felt guilty at first because I knew how it felt to be in her position. But Sally took it all very coolly. Once it was in the open, she was willing to accept it.

In December, Sally went abroad to spend Christmas in India. While she was away, I was more than happy to occupy her side of their bed. When I moved in temporarily with Fred, I was surprised to discover that he was a very religious Jew. Although he wasn't above matters of the flesh, he kept the Sabbath sacred. This meant that he wouldn't go out on Friday nights. I enjoyed helping him prepare a big dinner, and, especially, consuming large amounts of Sabbath wine. It was the only way Fred could get me to stay in on a Friday night. That and an evening of passionate lovemaking.

Still vulnerable, I found myself without a therapist to discuss my inner workings. After Daniel and I had finally broken up, my old psychologist (the same one who'd been so embarrassed about my spanking fantasies) showed no kind of reaction. He seemed to have no compassion. I soon stopped seeing him and luckily discovered a man named Walter Black. It was a pleasant change. Not only was Walter more caring, but he was totally interactive with me. With his help, I began to see that Fred possessed a narcissistic personality. As an emotional masochist, I was his perfect foil. Walter told me that narcissists attract masochists like moths to a flame. Narcissists think very highly of themselves and have little compassion for others. As a masochist, I traditionally picked men who put me down and were unobtainable. There was always a constant sense of pain, of longing. I had transferred much of the suffering and sense of loss I was feeling since Daniel had left me to Fred. Fred became one more hurt to wash away with alcohol, one more reason to get comfortably numb.

Fred had done one good thing, however. He convinced me that I could lecture at singles groups. Through this, my client base expanded from mostly women to some men. One of them was Al, a very uptight guy contemplating divorce. I began to counsel his wife too, then see them together. Vivacious and fun, I saw her blossom as she grew stronger. Eventually they decided to go their separate ways. I was fulfilled in knowing that I'd helped her, but a bit jealous that she had the strength to do something I never could—to leave a relationship that had died.

Normally, it would have taken me about two years to accumulate three thousand hours of service for my license, but with all of my activities, I was filling the requirement quickly. I still saw patients at Fred's office, discussing case histories with him. I was helping other people, but I seemed unable to help myself out of the destructive relationship with Fred. Because I was so screwed up mentally, I couldn't believe that I was able to help others. But the evidence was there. Some of my patients were getting well and would stop seeing me. This made me glad, but I couldn't help feeling abandoned as well.

In the end I couldn't deny how terribly the relationship with Fred was affecting me. I finally broke it off. I got another supervisor and started seeing clients out of my apartment. I began feeling very alone. Again.

I wasn't looking for anybody serious. After Fred, I was done in emotionally. I had no real goals in life except surviving. When I started seeing Fred I stopped going to the Queen Mary. With Fred gone I flew into that club with a frenzy. Somehow those one-night stands never bothered me. It seemed that the dancers were built for one-night stands. I didn't even want them to stay until morning. Just do it and leave. One time a man in a singles bar told me that I looked lost. Before I knew it I was back at his place. This was before AIDS, so I never worried about anything, except maybe herpes. There was cocaine. I never did it in those days unless it was free. I vaguely recall doing all sorts of uninhibited acts with that guy, whose name I can't even remember now—things you shouldn't do with a virtual stranger. When I woke up the next morning and took a good look at him, I was instantly repulsed. How could I have ended up with him?

The dancer's lifestyle seemed very attractive. I was lured by the idea of commercialized sex. Watching them disrobe to a cheering audience, I wondered if I could do it. Dollar bills were oozing out of their jock straps. What a fun way to make a living!—acting sexual, teasing. What the hell, I was acting sexual anyway and not getting paid for it. Could I shake my tits at strange, appreciative men? There was nothing to stop me now.

I envied the dancers' lives. I became a part of the scheme of things when I took one home with me. After watching those firm asses, those thick, flaccid dicks all night, I was pretty horny. I'd want one of them. Any one. Sam. Steven. It didn't matter who. Women lined up to talk to them. Other women wanted them. It was a thrill when one of them chose me to share his bed. It was like I'd won a prize or something.

Walking into the bathroom at the Queen Mary one night, I noticed a bunch of women huddled around a lady who frequented the club. Cathy had just admitted that she'd been raped a few nights before in the parking lot of another strip club called "Filthy McNasty's." There I was, rape counselor to the rescue. We talked a bit and exchanged phone numbers. Not only did I want to help Cathy, but I was glad to have found a buddy who enjoyed the male dancers as much as I did. My graduate school friends wouldn't be found dead in a place like the Queen Mary. Cathy had a very pretty face, but she was extremely overweight. I soon learned that we had a lot more than a rape experience in common. Cathy loved to drink and fuck as much as I did. She also enjoyed the challenge of bedding down the male strippers, so we frequented all of the clubs together. Cathy had been at it longer than I had. I was in for quite an education.

One night, Cathy had an interesting proposition. She had a couple of friends who wanted to meet me. Ernie and Raul were a pair of businessmen who owned a movie supply company in Burbank. Because they were married they restricted their partying schedule to special occasions. These were times when champagne and cocaine flowed freely. The usual scenario was that Cathy would get high and fuck them both, but Ernie kept asking her to get a friend to join in on the fun and games. Me. Cathy assured me that they fucked much better than any of the dancers. We set aside a night for a casual meeting. An innocent drink, I thought. Raul couldn't make it so Ernie's brother-in-law, Lon, was eager to fill in. They had a room at the Howard Johnson's right off the Hollywood Freeway. The very thought of this encounter excited me. It certainly seemed nasty and daring.

Dressed in a pair of black leotards and a baggy, striped shirt, I certainly looked like a fresh ingénue. I felt more like a hooker on a call. The guys had already been partying when I arrived. They weren't what I'd expected. They were in their early forties, definitely not male stripper types. Lon was an ugly, weathered version of Paul McCartney and didn't appeal to me in the least. Almost immediately he was grabbing my ass and tits. Ernie and Cathy were already busy kissing. Ernie was a bit younger than Lon and I found him adorable. There was cocaine all over the room. I snorted a few lines to catch up with the rest of them. Pretty soon I was feeling no pain, but no matter how high I got I didn't want to be with Lon. I whispered my dissatisfaction to Cathy and within minutes Lon was gone.

There we were, Ernie, Cathy, and me in a hotel room full of coke and chilled champagne. Ernie took me in his arms and began kissing me very passionately. I loved the feel of his tongue in my mouth and was giving in to it, loosening up. Suddenly, I felt a warm wetness on my pussy. It was Cathy lapping and sucking my clit. Now I understood why she wasn't possessive with her men—she liked women too. It probably turned her on to watch me with her boyfriend. Numbed by cocaine, I was having my first sexual experience with a woman. It was a very odd feeling. I kept trying to convince myself that it didn't really make any difference. What did it matter as long as it felt good? The drugs enabled me to tolerate almost anything, even something I found repulsive. I can't say I didn't enjoy the *ménage à trois,* but sex with more than one person is strangely less intimate.

Ernie left us about one in the morning to go home to his wife. The thought of being alone with Cathy left me in a state of momentary panic. I was worried that she would want to continue having sex with me. Luckily, she didn't. Instead, we ordered up breakfast and spent the night giggling like a couple of teenage girls at a slumber party. I left the next morning, but Cathy stayed on another night, thoroughly enjoying running up Ernie's bill and ordering room service whenever it caught her fancy.

After that night, Cathy decided to initiate three-ways with some of the dancers. Since there were only five men to a roomful of willing ladies, Cathy and I deduced that we would be more "marketable" if we teamed up. Most men entertain the fantasy of having two women at the same time, and we were more than willing to give them the luxury. Although I wasn't into women, I was very agreeable to the thought of sharing the cock of one of the dancers with Cathy. Steven and Sal were usually ripe for the picking if we caught them in the mood. I especially liked Steven. He was tall and beautifully built and had a "dick that wouldn't quit," to quote Cathy. A few times we managed to seduce both Steven and Sal together. The sex and the drugs would go on all night, starting off with a sensuous strip, courtesy of us ladies. One night Cathy and I simultaneously treated Steven to a juicy blow job in the middle of a park near the club in North Hollywood. There was nothing we wouldn't do, nothing we wouldn't sample in our endless quest for pleasure. Another time, Cathy begged me to have a threesome with a guy she'd been seeing. I couldn't understand it. How could she bear to share a man she really cared about with me? Something like that would drive me crazy. But it aroused Cathy to no end, appealing to both sides of her bisexual nature.

Thanksgiving that year wasn't the traditional turkey and dressing spread. Cathy and I had champagne and cocaine, then cruised down Santa Monica Boulevard to look at the sexy little male prostitutes. Wild with talk of seduction, we wound up at the Queen Mary. Even though it wasn't male stripper night, we sat through the transvestite show. Anything that smacked of sex was fine with us. After seeing the movie *Risky Business,* we decided that we wanted to have an adventure too. On the way home we picked up a hitchhiker and tumbled with him in the back seat of my car. He couldn't believe his good fortune. A ride and two women. A tumble of clothing. A tangle of zippers. Cathy was grinning. She did anything she craved, and that's why I liked her. She dared to do what I always wanted to, and now I was doing it, too.

Somehow, through all of this, I was still able to keep up my practice. It was like living a double life, being the dutiful, caring therapist and living a *Looking for Mr. Goodbar* existence at night. In my straight life during the day I was conferring with eight or ten regular clients a week. None of them was too sick. They were what I like to refer to as "normal neurotics." Most of them happened to be female. I really enjoyed seeing one, Debbie. Working as a secretary, she was in her late twenties. Basically she just wanted to talk about the men in her life, plus past and future relationships. One night, after I had seen her once a week for a couple of months, she really shocked me. Debbie told me that she had fantasies about being spanked. "You too?" I wanted to blurt out, ecstatically, relieved. It was the first time anyone had ever revealed that they had the same desires as I had to be spanked. Before Debbie, this fantasy had been unreal, like the far-out stuff you read about in magazines. The few times I dared to mention it to Daniel, or to my old therapist, the responses had been disastrous. I was convinced that no one ever felt the way I did. Certain that the idea of being turned on by spanking was sick and deviant, I was actually startled when Debbie began discussing it so easily.

Debbie told me she had met an Israeli and explained her crazy idea to him. He agreed to spank her, but later she got embarrassed and changed her mind. Months passed and she picked up an L.A. newspaper called the *Free Press.* It offered all kinds of sexual services. I didn't realize newspapers like that existed. I knew that the next day I would most certainly buy a copy. Debbie had actually gotten brave enough to phone one of the guys who had placed a spanking ad, but she lost her nerve and hung up when he answered the phone. Listening to her revelations, I wanted to tell her that I really understood. I wanted to be spanked and to be submissive with a man, too. But a therapist never should disclose her personal feelings. She should always be an objective listener. When Debbie told me about her fantasies, I could feel my face flushing. I was uncomfortable and embarrassed. In therapist's lingo, when you relate too closely to a client's problem, it's called "counter-transference." Debbie was definitely pressing my sex button, all right.

The following night I had no patients and was sitting at home alone. Ernie phoned me. Since his friend Raul still wanted to meet me, they wanted to come by my apartment and get acquainted. I said yes, but immediately called Cathy for emotional and physical support. Although she couldn't come and join the three of us, she had a suggestion. "Fuck them both," Cathy told me matter-of-factly. "I always do." To relax, I took a Quaalude. Ernie and Raul arrived with a couple of bottles of cheap champagne. I had the impression we were going to make a wild night of it, but it was only a brief stop. They were on their way home to their wives. Stoned, horny, and faced with the prospect of being alone all night, my clitoris was throbbing. I *had* to have sex. I dragged Ernie into my bedroom. Raul politely declined, anxious to get home to his wife, who was waiting with spaghetti and meatballs she'd made from scratch. In two minutes flat, Ernie shot off on my belly. I didn't have half a chance to reach a climax. Off in the living room, Raul was groaning that he had to leave. I begged Ernie to stay and finish me off. But he shrugged and kissed me on the forehead. Ernie's wife was waiting, too.

Still high and still horny, I didn't know what to do with myself. Then I remembered Debbie's casual mention of the *Free Press*. I rushed out and bought the latest edition, plus a bag of corn nuts to munch on. Seeing all of those ads about spanking—spanking—right there in newsprint was too much to bear. I pulled down my panties and made myself come in record time right there on the living room floor. Panting in the aftershock of my orgasm, I realized that it was still early. There I was, still horny and still with nothing to do. I was sure that a night at home with a bag of corn nuts wasn't what I craved.

I didn't know who I was calling. I didn't know exactly what I was getting into or what I was looking for. But very quickly I learned. Most of the large display ads were placed by bondage houses advertising their wares—spankings, dominants, submissives. Although I wan't quite sure what most of that was, I knew one thing. Females probably worked in those places and I certainly wasn't interested in being spanked by a woman. Only one ad offered the services of a man, but with my luck, he wasn't on call that night. Did I want to make an appointment? Hell, no. I wanted it *now!* Other places offered phone sex, but their manner was curt. I called yet another number. The first thing the woman on the line asked was my credit card number. I didn't have one. All of Daniel's and my credit cards had been destroyed after the divorce.

"Are you dominant or submissive?" she wanted to know.

These were new words for me.

"A submissive . . . I think," I told her.

When she asked me what I was into, I politely thanked her for her time and said I'd call back the next day. But I knew I wouldn't. Ready to give up, I suddenly read an ad that really intrigued me. "Sir William orders his slave Aurora to find submissive ladies to serve me. Couples OK. Never a fee." I must admit the "Never a fee" attracted me. The phone rang a number of times. Just as I was about to hang up, someone answered it.

"Yes," a male voice said, most authoritatively. Not "Hello," but "Yes."

Very timidly, I asked, "Could you explain what your ad means?"

"Well, if you don't know," he said, "then forget it." And he actually hung up on me!

Most people would have quit right then and there, but I guess the masochist in me persisted. I tried a few more calls, but all of them were the same—bondage houses looking for credit card numbers. I was so desperate that I decided to call Sir William again. He must have recognized my voice. "What do you want?" he asked tiredly. I stuttered and stammered, trying to explain that I had a fantasy, but was afraid to talk about it. Suddenly his voice softened. Not wanting him to hang up on me again, I took a deep breath and blurted out, "I've always wanted to get spanked." Breathlessly, I added, "I know it's crazy." The voice on the other end of the line chuckled. "Oh, is that all? That's not so crazy." Didn't he know how terrifying it was for me to even utter the word "spank" to another human being? Didn't he know that I thought I was perverted, deviant? Didn't he know that I'd be shunned by society if it knew? Sir William began to talk to me. All of the rudeness and gruffness was gone. This was a man who empathized with my fantasy, who understood. I sighed with relief. His response soothed me like going to the doctor and discovering I had a nasty twenty-four-hour virus and not cancer.

Suddenly I was telling Sir William how I dreamed of having a big, strong man drape me over his knees like a little girl. He would be forceful, sensual, and handsome. I was sure that if he spanked me the right way, we'd have incredible sex afterward.

"Do you want to get off over the phone?" he asked.

"No," I said quickly. "I want . . ."

"You want to be spanked," William growled sexily. He described himself as tall, dark, handsome and twenty-nine years old. He sounded like my dream man. He was also a Master. It was another new word, but I was sure I'd discover what it was.

William lived about twenty minutes away, in Glendale. We agreed to meet in a nearby coffeeshop and talk first. To put me more at ease, William added, "Meeting me this way is a lot safer than picking up a stranger in a bar." It made perfect sense to me. My curiosity was piqued and I was ripe for adventure. My adrenalin was pumping hard. I pulled into the empty parking lot more excited than nervous. The coffeeshop was closed, but William was standing there waiting for me. Immediately I knew he wasn't my type. From his description, I was expecting a virile, muscular motorcycle man dripping in black leather. William looked like an accountant with thick, dark-rimmed glasses. He was probably closer to forty than his professed twenty-nine. I wanted to leave on the spot, but decided it would do no harm just to talk. After all, I'd come this far.

My state of mind went from hard dick to flaccid. Disappointed, I followed William to a nearby coffeeshop. The small talk didn't last very long. Very friendly, William explained that he had been a part of the S&M scene for years. "So, you've always wanted to be spanked," he smiled. How did he know? Did it show that much? Next came a question about my childhood. He wondered if my parents had spanked me as a little girl. The last thing I wanted to do was discuss my abusive mother. "Let's just talk sexy," I thought. William must have picked up on this from my silence. He began to discuss spanking again. Just hearing the word "spank" made me melt. To this day, it isn't merely the physical act that arouses me so intensely. Like Pavlov's dog, whenever I hear that word, I'm immediately turned on. As we talked my whole body began to shake. My voice raced like a quivery undercurrent as I began to discuss my most hidden secret with a virtual stranger. For the first time in my life I was actually speaking freely and honestly about being spanked. It was also the first time that my listener understood exactly what I was talking about.

William let me babble on. Finally I fell silent. "You are a true submissive lady," he told me. There was that word again. I still wasn't sure what it meant. But William went on to explain. "You have a real need to be told what to do. You hate making decisions. Deep down, you don't really know how to take care of yourself. You're happiest when you're serving a man. And you like the feeling of being overpowered and helpless."

How did William know all of my secrets? Even though I knew he wasn't my dream man, all of this talk aroused me to new heights. I wanted to be spanked more than ever. I soon discovered that William was heavily into the S&M lifestyle. As a Master, when he was with a woman, she had to be submissive, his slave. Right then and there he convinced me that I was really a true submissive. The more he talked, the more convincing it sounded. "You need a man in your life who will tell you what to do and give you direction," William insisted. This grated against my sensibilities as a feminist, but made sense in many ways. I'd felt so lost since Daniel had left. I knew I needed something, but I wasn't certain what it was. I wanted someone to mold me and arouse me sexually at the same time.

William made being a submissive sound like such a positive thing. Smiling, he told me that he'd never met anyone with as much potential as I had. "I could take you home," he said, "put you over my knee and just spank you. But there's much more to you than that, Alice." I wanted to go off with William. I wanted to get spanked. But there were many questions. Would he lead me back to the freeway when it was over? Would he leave marks on my body? Would he hurt me? As we walked out the door, I suddenly turned to William and asked, "But I haven't been bad or done anything wrong. Why am I being spanked?" William's eyes lit up. "Oh, so you need a reason." He thought for a moment. "What do you think your friends would say if they knew you'd answered an ad in a sleazy newspaper, met the guy, and gone home with him to get spanked? Do you think they'd say you were a bad girl?"

I didn't know what to say.

"I'm sure they'd agree that a sound spanking is exactly what you deserved, Alice."

My legs were shaking as we went to our cars. Perhaps I looked as frightened as I felt.

"Don't worry," William assured me. "I'll take good care of you."

8

Spanked

The roads twisted up the hills that overlooked Los Angeles. With my awful sense of direction, I was sure I'd get lost on the way back down to the freeway. But at least my ass would be pleasantly tingly from the spanking I was going to receive from Sir William. We finally arrived. William lived in a very scary, remote location. Actually, it was a one-bedroom shack. William could have murdered me and buried me in the front yard and no one would ever have known. It looked like Charles Manson's summer place. Here I was, anxious to go inside with a strange man to fulfill an insane sexual fantasy.

The telephone was ringing when we came through the door. William told me to sit and wait until he was finished. I could hear him describing me to his caller. "Yeah," he chuckled, "I have a cute little blonde here just waiting to get spanked. She's waiting here so patiently in a pretty pink jumpsuit." I could tell that he was talking to another woman, because William asked about her Master. They sounded as though they were members of some secret society. I later learned that William had been speaking to Martin and Marlene, a couple very much into S&M. Marlene was a total slave who wore rings through her pierced nipples. It all sounded barbaric, totally dark and evil. William told me that Martin forced Marlene to walk around naked wearing only a pair of very high-heeled shoes. All I could think of was how uncomfortable it must have been. It didn't seem very sexy to me, since I liked to bounce around my apartment barefoot and in an old t-shirt. Trudging naked in stiletto heels was a bit too bizarre for me. That wasn't my trip at all. What I wanted was a little girl spanking, not a journey into another dimension.

Oddly enough, Martin and Marlene's relationship gave me the same feelings I got when I first read *The Story of O,* which is a sort of bible to people involved with S&M. It is the tale of one woman's total love for a man. O is so obsessed with him that she allows him to take her to a place called "Roissy," where she is kept as a willing prisoner. She's forced to wear clothing that makes both her front and rear accessible to any man who wants to sample her. O is chained at night and beaten each day by a valet. Later, her lover gives her to his mentor, an older man. Although O doesn't like him at first, she obeys him to please her lover, to show what a good slave she is. Eventually she falls in love with the mentor. The whippings fascinated me, but the rest left me feeling somewhat revolted and confused about feminist teachings. My mind wandered through thoughts of O as William finished speaking on the phone.

I was actually expecting an amiable chat from William before we began. Suddenly, his face turned grim and his eyes became steely. "Take off your clothes," he ordered.

"What?" I gasped in a frightened voice.

"You heard me," William said.

Something in his tone told me it wouldn't be wise to disobey. Unbuttoning my jumpsuit, I slowly let it fall to the ground. William pushed me against the wall, told me to spread my legs and assume a policeman's frisking stance. Legs apart, my hands were stretched above me. William slowly ran his hand along my body. He wasn't being sexual, because I'd made it clear at the restaurant that I didn't want to make love with him, only to be spanked.

Very soon, William was smacking my ass with his open palm. It didn't hurt at all. After ten swats, it still didn't sting. Actually, it felt rather pleasant—but it wasn't exactly what I desired. I wanted William to be an angry daddy or boyfriend. The role-playing aspect was important to me. Today, I can peg my desires as "corporal punishment," which is very specific and different from your standard S&M. It's not so much that the man or woman wants to be submissive. Rather, they want to enact a little scene. My desire was very specialized and William was engulfed in S&M in general.

But I had to obey. For some reason, William wanted me to address him as "Sir." He also instructed me to say "Thank you, sir," after each blow. Although I felt as though I were a member of King Arthur's Court, I complied. As the night wore on, William had me assume many different spanking positions. On all fours. Kneeling over a chair. Flat on my stomach. Sprawled over an ottoman—his personal favorite. He instructed me to count and then thank him after each blow. "One, thank you, sir . . . two, thank you, sir . . ." I felt like a student immersed in studying "S&M 101." William's game was more psychological. I was getting tired of counting.

I felt almost as though I were an observer watching the scene. Why didn't William understand what I really wanted? Why was he calling me a slut, a bitch, and a whore? What was the point of all this "sir" stuff? We played games for hours and hours. William even made me lick his shoes. "Whose dog-bitch are you?" he demanded.

"I'm yours, sir," I told him meekly.

"Say it!"

"Yes, sir, I'm yours."

"And what are you?"

"I'm your slut, sir. I'm your slave, sir."

At first I felt a bit guilty because William had agreed to spank me. But it wasn't long before I realized that I was enacting his favorite fantasy. He wasn't doing me a favor at all. I was unwittingly contributing to his verbal humiliation/female dog trip. All I wanted was a simple spanking and I wasn't getting much of that. Not that the experience was entirely unpleasant, but it hadn't progressed the way I'd hoped. William kept at it for three hours. I really think he assumed he was turning me on, but actually I felt ambivalent. William was sitting on the sofa observing my crouched form across the room. "What position does slave wish to assume next?" he asked.

"I want to lie across your knees," I told him.

Finally he said, "All right, *slave.*" ("Why is he calling me that?" I kept wondering.) "Crawl across the room and drape yourself over my lap."

Crawl . . . drape. The very words aroused me. Slowly, I moved toward him. As soon as I knew he could see my bare ass, totally vulnerable, I became incredibly excited. Lying across a man's lap is really a very sexy position because your crotch is in direct contact with his knee. The friction on the vulva and clit is compounded by the impact of the smacks. For me, it was a total physical and mental arousal.

Holding my ass upward, I hungrily met each of William's blows. Savoring each smack, I felt I could stay there forever. The turn-on for me was in being admonished, punished. It also was the thought of being forced over a man's lap. I wasn't particularly aroused by the thought of pain itself. That's what most people have so much difficulty understanding. Not the pain, but the *anticipation* of the administering of pain. When you're extremely aroused, your brain turns pain into pleasure. William didn't try to touch me between the legs. He just kept spanking and I kept wiggling. Finally, he stopped and told me to get up.

Taking a breather, we sat and smoked cigarettes, talking about the experience. That was an interesting thing about William. While he could get immersed in role-playing, he was a very understanding friend and a good listener when the games were over. "Tell me how you feel right now," he said.

"I'm really glad that it finally happened," I admitted. "I've wanted to be spanked for as long as I can remember. But I don't know how I'm going to feel tomorrow. Will I hate myself in the morning?" I was already thinking ahead to the date I had the next night with a very straight ex-lover from college. And would I dare tell my shrink about this experience? It was as though I'd stepped over the line of "socially acceptable" behavior. I'd finally had the courage to explore that deep, dark, secret part of myself. But how would I ever reconcile this masochistic need with the other, "straight" areas of my life? Part of me felt relieved, but another part felt ashamed. We talked for almost an hour. All the while William tried to get me to feel proud about "coming out of the closet." He told me how good I was, what an incredible spanking I could endure, trying his best to turn my negative feelings into positive ones. "You're such a natural submissive," he stressed. I'd never felt "natural" about anything in my life. Anything I achieved, I had had to work damned hard for.

William gave me the freedom to come down and visit him whenever I felt the need. No wonder William felt so strongly about what I'd done. I later learned how intensely he believed that the dominant/submissive relationship is the best way of life. At the 1990 "Lifestyles" convention in Las Vegas (an event that celebrates alternative lifestyles), William watched a couple playing an S&M game with each other. The woman's Master tapped her lightly with his whip as she conversed with other people. "If she were *my* slave," William pontificated, "I wouldn't

let her talk to anyone. She'd stand there silently with her head down."
How absurd, I thought. This was a party. People were here to have
fun. Nevertheless, that's the way he felt a slave should act and that's
the way he taught me to act. I think it's fine to play whatever sex
games you wish. That's the beauty of it—there doesn't have to be any
rules. S&M shouldn't be taken so deathly seriously. There are no such
things as real slaves or real Masters in this world. All of us are equals.
You can choose to play the game as seriously as you wish, but you
have to come back to reality. S&M isn't the real world.

Originally Sir William tried to lead me down a very different path.
He's the most serious "Master" I've ever encountered during the eight
years I've been involved in S&M. He groomed me to be a submissive
and I was ripe for it. Look how obediently I followed him to his house
that first night. Thinking back, it's too bad that my first encounter
wasn't with someone who was more lighthearted about the whole scene.
At first I didn't ever question William. I was afraid of him, uncertain
what he would do next, and fear can be an aphrodisiac. I did have
a choice, though—to be trained as William's private slave, or to use
his place as an occasional pleasure den.

Talking with William so honestly made me feel much better. It
was only a year after Daniel and I had split up and I was still feeling
very vulnerable. Working hard toward taking my licensing exam, I was
mentally exhausted. William couldn't have come into my life at a better time. I stopped running around and trying to seduce guys, because
now I had another outlet. William made me feel better about the person I was. I suddenly realized that plenty of other people shared my
fantasies. But since we'd met through an ad in a sex tabloid, sometimes I couldn't believe he was a real person.

That first night we must have talked until four or five in the morning. William was willing to spank me again before I left, but I was
still very horny.

"I think I should go home and masturbate," I confessed.

"No problem," William told me. "I can get you off right here."

Although I still felt very strongly about our "no sex" agreement,
I couldn't refuse his offer. William fingered my burning pussy so ex-
quisitely that I had the quickest, most violent climax I've ever had in
my life. He seemed surprised. "You really have a lot of untapped sexuality inside of you. Are you aware of the power this gives you?" Feeling sexually obligated toward William for fulfilling my fantasy, I took

his penis into my mouth. Much to my relief, it didn't take long for him to climax either. Before I left, William turned me over his knee one more time. I counted out the twenty resounding smacks. "One," I said happily, "thank you, sir. Two, thank you, sir." He finally sent me home with a warmly glowing behind.

Leading me to the freeway entrance, William made me promise I'd phone him to let him know I'd gotten home safely. I kept thinking of how sweet he was. No one had ever worried like that about me. Later, my therapist couldn't help chuckling. "So, you've met the world's most caring sadist. He sounds much nicer than any of the guys you've told me about so far!"

For the next few days, I was playing with myself continuously, reliving the scene over and over again in my head. I couldn't help thinking about lying across William's lap and pressing my clit against his knee. As I studied for the licensing exams, I took breaks to diddle myself. My therapist congratulated me for doing something I'd desired for such a long time. I had taken a wild risk by going off with a stranger, but, thankfully, it worked out in a positive way. At that point, I honestly felt that would be it. My evening with William would be a pleasant memory and I'd never have a spanking session again.

My ass was totally black and blue. (That commonly happens to spanking virgins.) It wasn't William's fault entirely, because I loved it. Every time he hit me, I kept raising up my ass to meet the blows. My date with Peter, my very straight college chum, was uneventful. He took me to an Amway meeting. What a turnabout! One night I was playing S&M games in a peculiar dungeon and the next I'm at a sales meeting. My biggest fear was that Paul would want to go to bed with me. I couldn't let him see my bruised behind.

I didn't see William that whole week. Masturbating to my memories was more than sufficient. But soon I found myself digging out the old newspaper and thumbing through for William's number, "just to say hello," I kept thinking as I dialed his number. William praised me for being such a good submissive. I needed to hear that I was competent at something and that someone really appreciated me. He gave my feelings a name and he gave them a place where they could be expressed. Not only was I a "submissive," but I was an excellent one! That probably explained why I had never been aggressive or assertive. I needed a strong man to guide me. A submissive person chooses to do these things anyway, but the Dominant gives them the strength, the reason to be as they are. As a shy exhibitionist, I was "forced" to perform certain acts that I really wanted to do anyway. My fantasy had been that someone would come along and do this for me. It was a new twist on the old knight-in-shining-armor daydream. I wouldn't have to seek this man out. Somehow he would find me. If I were being cranky, plagued by PMS, or bitchy, this dream Dominant would take me over his knee and spank me. He wouldn't walk out the door or ignore me like Daniel did. This man would truly love me. William wasn't that dream man, but he helped me realize that I didn't have to be fearful anymore. I could stand up on my own two feet as long as I had someone to guide me and protect me from the rest of the world.

I was too embarrassed to tell any of my college friends about the enactment of my fantasy. Eventually I told Laura about Marlene and her pierced nipples. She equated it with mutilating the female body. The only person I received any sort of encouragement from was Cathy. And that happened almost by accident. It was about two weeks after my encounter with William. Cathy had stopped by my place and we were planning to go out that night. She was changing her clothes in front of me and I couldn't help but notice the florid bruises that decorated her ass.

"Cathy, what happened?" I asked in disbelief.

She fumbled around for an answer. "Oh, I fell down some stairs," she told me.

I knew Cathy was lying, but she wouldn't admit where she'd gotten those marks. This was my chance to open up with another woman. I was dying to tell her about what I'd experienced with William. When Cathy promised not to tell a soul, I described my entire evening with Sir William in delicious detail. Cathy's eyes were wide with interest. She didn't laugh as I'd feared. "Oh, Alice," she said dreamily, "I just have to meet him." As it turned out, those welts on Cathy's behind were from sex games she had played with her cousin. Sometimes he'd beat her with his belt and she just loved it. I couldn't believe my ears when she elaborated on their antics. "Sometimes he ties me up and hangs me naked from a rafter. As I'm dangling there helpless, he beats my ass." I wanted to meet her cousin, but first Cathy begged me to phone Sir William so we could visit him for an S&M adventure. I finally gave in and called William. Luckily, he was home. It seemed as though he was always there, a mysterious voice on the other end of the line, endlessly waiting.

William seemed intrigued at the prospect of having two slaves at his mercy and he gave me explicit instructions. The both of us were to dress very sexily in hot pants and tank tops. We had to paint our fingernails a bright, slutty red. "Be here at eight o'clock sharp, or else," he warned, making it all too obvious that bad things would happen to us if we were late. Cathy was very excited, but I was jittery, wondering why I was going back.

On the way to our meeting place, I became customarily lost. Because of that, we were a bit late. Sir William was fuming, and I was certain he'd punish us for our tardiness. He ordered me to sit in the seat beside him. Cathy followed us close behind, driving my car. Alone with him, William asked me about Cathy. I told him all I knew, how we'd met at the Queen Mary. How Cathy was always horny.

The moment we stopped outside of his dilapidated house, William became our Master. His voice was stern and his eyes were cold. He ushered Cathy into the house while I was ordered to wait in the locked car with my head between my legs. I was being punished for my lateness. As I sat there docile, I wondered how he was punishing Cathy. I did exactly as William told me. I waited and waited. It seemed like hours. That's part of the turn-on, I suppose. The air of mystery. The air of anticipation. Cathy and I had a lot of fun just dressing and preparing for this episode. We did our makeup meticulously and painted each other's nails. By the time we were done, we were feeling like nasty little tramps—a very good reason to get punished. One of the most important aspects in a dominant/submissive relationship is to have absolute trust in your Master. Although I didn't know William very well, I was sure he wasn't insane, that he would never really hurt me.

Finally, he came out and led me into the house. I beheld a sight I couldn't believe. Cathy was on all fours, stark naked, leashed, and collared. She was blindfolded and had a big gag in her mouth. Breasts dangling, three clothespins were clamped onto each nipple. She looked like a freak, like some grotesque, wild animal. "What do you think of your friend now?" William asked, obviously proud of his handiwork.

I started a long, babbling speech of protest. "You can't do this," I yelled at William. "This is terrible. You don't understand. This girl was raped recently. You're going to really fuck her up . . . ."

William was laughing at my naiveté. He took the gag out of Cathy's mouth. "Go ahead. Tell her, Cathy. Tell Alice how you feel."

"Oh, Alice, I'm in heaven," Cathy moaned with pleasure.

Okay, I thought. All right. I was beginning to understand. This was the world of sadomasochism. There was no turning back now. Leaving Cathy with her ass in the air, William grabbed me, yanked up my skirt, pulled down my panties, and put me over his knee. I got spanked. This time I screamed because he was really hurting me. I wasn't high or drunk and I wasn't very aroused. William seemed very pleased dividing his attentions between Cathy and myself, whipping Cathy, then spanking me, yelling at the both of us for our disobedience. It was definitely his own trip, not ours. William forced me into the basic slave position— down on the knees, legs spread apart. Crouching naked at his feet, I had to kiss his shoes and worship his very existence.

Over and over again, Cathy and I repeated this little performance. We did whatever William told us to. I noticed that he was much rougher with Cathy than with me, more physically abusive. Cathy was his bondage queen, his champion of nipple torture. With me, William applied more verbal humiliation. In between his strict orders, there was lots of spanking. He kept dropping his shoe on the floor and making me retrieve it with my mouth.

Finally, giggling, I looked at him and said, "This is like dog training."

William laughed. "Exactly. You're my dog-bitch." Fortunately, although William was a serious Master, he also had a sense of humor. Unlike other Masters and Mistresseses, he "allowed" laughter when a situation became funny or absurd.

After that episode, I became more heavily involved with William. He wanted me to call him every night at eleven. I liked the idea of having someone to report to, someone who was looking out for me. About that time of night, I often found myself feeling very lonely. Soon we were doing phone fantasies together. William would have me tell him stories about humiliation. He was amazed that someone like me, who had no knowledge of the S&M scene, could always be right on target.

"I am in a room," I would tell William, "totally naked, surrounded by men. They all want me. They're so hot. They stand around me in a circle as I lie there on my back, legs spread wide apart."

"How do you feel?" William would ask.

"I feel like a bad little girl. I am the only woman in the room. These men are stroking their cocks until they grow nice and hard and I love watching them. I spread my pussy lips so they can see how pink I am inside."

"Are you wet?" William's voice would groan.

"Very wet," I would tell him. "I want them to fuck me, all of them.

But they don't. I've been a bad girl, so they torment me with their cocks. No one will touch me, so I just touch myself."

I could tell that William was stroking his own cock as he spoke to me. "And then what?"

"I am their cum receptacle. One by one, these men shoot on me," I would whisper sexily. "One by one, they spurt their hot jism all over my body. I rub it into my skin. Sticky. Frothy. Then another man shoots his load onto me. Then another, until I'm covered with sperm from head to toe."

In a voice raspy with lust, William would praise me for bringing my Master off in an explosive climax using words. He often asked me to tell him stories about myself being with another slave. Closing my eyes, I could recount the events as though they were actually occurring. The female slave and I would get along very well because both of us would be trying to please our Masters. Sometimes we'd whip each other for their viewing pleasure. Like Scheherazade, I was conjuring up stories to please my Master. William was training me to be obedient, and I wanted to make him happy in any way I could. I was the good little girl and he was my daddy, making me feel protected and warm. I needed his praise and began to thrive on it.

I was surprised to find that I was feeling sexually attracted to William. A few weeks after our first three-way visit, Cathy and I went to see William again.

"Am I permitted to love my Master?" I asked William when we were alone.

"Yes, it often happens," he said rather blandly. The way William saw it, we weren't two people, but two roles.

That night, I craved to spend some time alone with William. He was keeping Cathy and me in separate rooms and running back and forth between us. Trying to get more attention, Cathy was playing the obstinate child. Constantly snapping out of her slave role, she actually yelled at William. After he'd scolded her sufficiently, he'd come into my room and amuse himself with me.

"What are you?" William asked.

"I am a slave, sir."

"What else are you?"

"I am a bitch. A slut. A whore. Scum. Slime. Trash, sir." The things I said just to get spanked!

At one point, William took off his shoes. It was my duty to lick his feet, something I really didn't like. I made this known to my Master, but he took great delight in making me perform this duty to confirm my submissive nature. I didn't want William to lose his temper, because then he could get very nasty, dreaming up punishments right out of high school detention hall. Writing something like, "I must be a more obedient slave" hundreds of times, until you felt like your hand was going to drop off.

When William left me to tend to Cathy, I strained to hear what they were saying but couldn't. I was very glad when she finally fell asleep on his bed, exhausted. For some reason, I fantasized that our sexual encounter would be romantic and intimate, but reality often shatters fantasies to bits. William was about as sensual as a man jerking off in a porno booth. He was a hard-driving, fast fuck with no edge of gentleness, but at that moment I desired him so much that it felt good. I just needed more, perhaps his tongue on my cunt, to bring me over the edge. But it was all right. It was better than being alone.

After it was over, I was feeling relaxed and playful. Usually, after a dominant scene, it's all right to be just Alice and William and talk like friends. It was warm and cozy with him on the couch, my mind not set on being a slave or a dog. I was a woman being cuddled by a man she cared about. "What would you do if I ever wanted to spank or dominate you?" I innocently asked William, my buried dominant nature surfacing.

The peace of the moment was shattered like glass. William's eyes became smoky and penetrating. Suddenly he was snarling like a dog who had turned on its owner. "Don't you *ever* talk like that again. Don't even think of it," he warned. "The next time you do, I'm going to force you to wear this to publicly humiliate you." William held up a rubber pig mask for emphasis. He made it quite clear that I was never to forget who was the Master and who was the slave. Although I didn't bring it up again, another seed was planted.

After that night, Cathy decided to drop out of our scene. That estranged our friendship because I had become even more involved with William. I asked my Master's permission for everything. He gave me free rein, but instructed me to be home by eleven every evening to call him. One time Cathy and I were out at the Queen Mary. It was a lucky night, because we'd picked up Steven and Sal. I rushed off to my place to call William and Cathy promised to bring the strippers by later. They walked in just as William told me to put the telephone receiver between my legs and hump it for him.

After that first time, William rarely fucked me. My compulsion to visit him wasn't sexual, but a delicious combination of fear and excitement. I enjoyed the games we played together, especially the spanking. Good Dominants don't get mad, they get even! Hopefully, the punishment is creative enough to please both parties. For keeping my Master waiting on the telephone too long, my punishment was to be paddled. But since William didn't own a paddle, we took a little excursion to the "Pleasure Chest."

The Pleasure Chest was a store that had an extensive S&M section. Along with leather clothes, sexy greeting cards, lotions, and dildos, there were many sex toys to choose from. Not only had William instructed me to purchase a paddle to be punished with later, but I had to request that the salesman try out a few different ones on my behind. My Master also informed me how he wanted me to dress—in a tight miniskirt with white lace panties underneath. I was excited at the prospect of the visit. William also gave me permission to act like a slut, something I've always longed to do but never had the nerve. That's the way it is with many submissives—their Masters permit them to express things they've been hiding away inside of them.

I didn't spot William in the Pleasure Chest right away. In fact, when I did, I wasn't even supposed to acknowledge him. I found the S&M section upstairs. The paddles were encased behind a glass counter that also housed all sorts of things I'd never seen before. Nonetheless, I felt at home. The store was evidence that many others besides William and myself played S&M games. There must have been at least fifty kinds of cock rings and twenty-five varieties of nipple clamps. I felt William's eyes upon me, watching me, so I quickly set out upon my quest. There were so many paddles to choose from. To be honest, my own personal criterion was to find one that was the least painful. Being spanked was one thing, but being hit with an object was quite another.

I asked the salesman for some assistance. It seemed as normal as buying a watch. First he asked my price range. Did I want wood or leather, soft or hard, studded or not? I blushed, "One that doesn't hurt too much."

The salesman smiled. That narrowed my choice down to a pair of leather paddles reinforced with metal braces inside. "Metal?" I gasped.

"Much better than the floppy kind, dear," he told me. "The soft ones tend to mark."

The paddles were basically the same except for the shape. One was larger, big enough to swat two cheeks at once, while the other was more round and resembled a traditional ping-pong paddle. I didn't know how to make my choice and then explained my plight. "My Master ordered me to try out the paddles before I bought one," I confessed.

"Sorry, that's against the rules," the salesman said.

"But he's watching. I'll be punished if you don't paddle me," I explained in a desperate tone.

"I'd love to, but . . ."

William had schooled me well in begging and groveling. I employed my sexiest little-girl whine. "Please . . ."

The salesman finally relented and gave me a few mild smacks on the behind. People in the store were watching and my unflappable shopkeeper seemed a bit embarrassed, but he was bent on customer satisfaction. I decided on the smaller paddle and thanked him for his indulgence.

As I stood at the counter ready to pay for my purchase, William magically appeared. There was a big grin on his face, so I was certain I'd pleased him. I was elated. You see, all I ever wanted was to be a good girl. William was teaching me to be "good" in ways that society traditionally considered "bad." He quickly paid for the purchase, which was my reward. It was odd. For being a good girl, I was going to be rewarded with pain.

After our visit to the sex emporium, William took me on a grand tour of the seedier side of Los Angeles. The Pleasure Chest was located on Santa Monica Boulevard in Hollywood, a place where all the male hookers hang out. We discussed the prospect of renting a cute stud and having him watch me get paddled for the first time. "Maybe I'll even let one of them spank you," William conceded. But this was only a tease. We drove on. At Santa Monica and Western, William escorted me to Stan's Bookstore, which boasted the largest collection of S&M books and tapes in the city. It was the first time I'd been in a place like that, and I loved it. The slimy, seedy side of life really appealed to me. Again, I was amazed that there was so much published information on the subject. There were apparently hoards of other folks who loved to get their fannies pinkened. The evidence was all around me.

For years, my titillation was focused on haphazard discoveries of occasional spanking letters in mainstream magazines like *Penthouse*. I had
no idea there were books and publications that specialized on the subject.

After Stan's, we headed back west on Santa Monica. The boy William had considered hiring to spank me was no longer there, so we
continued on our journey. A few blocks later, we drove down a residential street on San Vincente. "Look over there," William said. He pointed
to a modest two-story building. "That's the Chalet."

The Chalet! I'd heard so much about that place. In my naiveté,
I'd expected a fancy neon sign outside a grand, castlelike building. Someone had once told me about the Chalet, casually mentioning that a
friend used to visit it regularly to get whipped. I tried to conceal my
shock. Did people actually do those things? I supposed they did.

I was a bit disappointed the Chalet didn't look more dramatic, like
Dracula's castle looming on a cliff in the old black-and-white movies.
But the idea of what went on it aroused me.

"I'll take you there sometime," William promised. "We'll rent a
dungeon."

"Can we go now?" I wanted to know.

"Not tonight. I have other things planned."

We ended up at the Star Strip on La Cienga, which was one of
my Master's favorite night spots. A connoisseur of male stripdom, I
was now in virgin territory. I was worried that the female dancers would
be giving me dirty looks if they saw me as competition, but the atmosphere
was quite different. Actually, they seemed to like having a woman in
the audience. This club featured something called "table dancing." There
were about six large, round tables in the club and each had a different
lady undulating on top of it. William gave me money to tip each of
them. They flirted with me and I flirted right back. I wasn't attracted
to women, but William had given me that sanction to be bad. Flirting
with women definitely qualified.

William had the fantasy that every woman was secretly into S&M.
That night, one of the dancers revealed black and blue marks on her
behind. William and I speculated about how they got there. He even
ordered me to tell a few people present that I was a slave and he my
Master. There were mild smiles and not a hint of surprise. Everyone
seemed to know what I was talking about. I felt comfortable with my
life. I belonged.

The tour of L.A.'s underground was topped off by going back to

William's place. Underneath my tight skirt I was wearing the sexy panties, garter belt, and stocking ensemble William had instructed me to purchase especially for that evening. It was a kind of clothing I'd never worn before. Because I'd grown up in the liberated sixties and seventies, I was weaned on the feminist ideal that lingerie was oppressive to women. Deep down, I felt they were expressive samples of our femininity. I was glad that my Master had "ordered" me to put on something I'd craved to wear for so many years.

Inspired by the strippers, I did my own private show for William. I felt incredibly sensual as I removed my clothing piece by piece and saw William watching me attentively. Part of his pleasure was probably in knowing that he was helping me liberate the pent-up sexuality he claimed I was teeming with. For that I was very grateful. William was showing me a side of human sexuality I had only read about, dreamed about. I was fascinated.

The paddle was not as scary as I had anticipated. Although I still preferred the contact of the human hand over the coolness of leather against my skin, the more intense fear and the texture of the material made the paddle a nice change of pace.

Much of William's and my sex still consisted of verbal stimulation. I would tell him a sexy story while he'd jerk off, then he'd tell me a spanking story to accompany my own masturbation. Occasionally I spent the night at his house. One evening William chained me naked to a bench. I was immobile for hours. To keep me in line, he swore that if I moved or made a sound, he'd have the disgusting drunk who lived next door fuck me. I never dared challenge him.

We also passed the time by skimming through the sex tabloids and answering some of the ads. William kept saying that he wanted us to get together with another couple. One of his favorite verbal fantasies involved a story where the two of us would get together with another Master/slave couple. The man would be very attractive and his submissive pretty, but not a threat to me. They would live in a gorgeous mansion in Beverly Hills. After William and I arrived, the slave and I would go off into another room while our Masters planned their strategy. After an hour or so, our Masters would come for us. Blindfolded, with our hands firmly cuffed behind our backs, they would lead us to the dungeon downstairs. I would be strung up beside the other slave and there would be a contest of sorts to see which woman could endure more pain. Then, each slave would have to suck the other Master's cock. The girl who made the Master climax first would be rewarded with having her pussy eaten to a violent climax by the other slave. By the time I reached the conclusion of this story, William's prick would be swollen and ready to spurt. I was always the one who could endure the most whipping in the tale. And although I didn't entertain lesbian fantasies, they obviously aroused my Master. I was only too happy to oblige. After all, I was a model slave.

Perhaps to transform this dream into reality, William instructed me to call another Master—Martin—one night. He sounded very sexy and handsome over the telephone, and I hoped his slave, Marlene, would be instructed to share him with me some day soon. "I want to know one thing," Martin asked. "Are you in love with Sir William, or are you in love with S&M?" The truth was that I was in love with the scene and not with my Master. I was in love with the freedom to express my sexuality in the form of S&M play. But, being an obedient slave, I told Martin what I knew he wanted to hear.

As it turned out, William and I never did meet with Martin and Marlene. I was a bit disappointed, because I craved contact with another slave. There was no one I could talk to about my submissive feelings. I'd hoped there'd be an instant camaraderie between Marlene and myself. Marlene was a secretary and she too lacked someone she could speak to "slave to slave." From what Martin told me, she was looking forward to the same kind of friendship. Because of my Master's arrogance, however, we never met. Marlene called one day and William instructed her to call back at a designated time. For some reason, she never did. "I never call back a slave," William explained to me. If she wasn't being submissive enough over the telephone, perhaps he thought, she'd be a waste of time in other capacities.

One day I arrived home to a message from my Master on my answering machine. This surprised me, because we only spoke at night. I didn't even have William's work number. My heart skipped a beat when I heard William's strong voice ordering me to phone someone named "Master Alex" as soon as I walked in the door. Alex and Terry were a suburban, working-class couple who lived in the Valley. Married for fifteen years, they even had a few children. The tape instructed me to take off all my clothing and kneel on the floor when I called Master Alex. I was to obey all of Master Alex's orders as though they were coming from William himself.

Alex's first question was whether I was wearing an ankle bracelet.

To symbolize their submission, slaves often wear ankle chains on the right leg. Since I didn't have that piece of jewelry, Alex had me tie a string around my ankle. There were other silly acts, such as humping the telephone and spanking myself while counting off the swats. Then Alex told me to crawl on all fours to the bathroom. After I licked the toilet bowl, I crawled back to the telephone and shouted, "I am a toilet-licking bitch," over and over again. Can you believe I did all of this? Since I knew Alex would give a full report to William, I wanted to be the kind of slave my Master would be proud of. After all, a good slave is living proof of her Master's training ability.

Later that night, I recounted the details of the phone session to William. Perhaps I was a bit too surly and smug for a slave as I criticized Alex's stilted domination techniques. But William would teach me a lesson. "I wanted you to see the difference between a good Master and a bad Master," William told me.

"Master Alex made me kiss the toilet," I told William. "But at least I didn't have to drink out of it." The moment the words left my mouth, I knew I'd made a mistake.

William's voice took on a rough edge. "Does that thought disgust you, slave?"

I was silent.

"I command you to go into the bathroom, pee into a cup and come back to the telephone."

I did just as my Master said.

"Now, take a sip," William continued.

I did. It tasted so disgusting that I spit it out and began to choke. But William was still pleased. I was a good slave. At least I'd done what I was told.

We finally met Alex and Terry at a fast-food restaurant in the Valley. To say that they were not an attractive couple is being very polite. Terry was grotesquely thin and had very short hair. Her loose, polyester dress did little to compliment her appearance. She had the worst teeth I'd ever seen. A few of them were even missing. Alex reminded me of a big, dumb lug you might see in an "Archie" comic book. He was brutish and didn't speak very politely to his wife. As we had dinner together, it occurred to me that Terry was an abused wife. They were trying to mask their violent marriage under the title of S&M, but, in truth, it was not a game. He was cruel to her. This fact bothered me. Real violence always upsets me. It's nothing like the consensual brand of play shared by people within the bounds of a bondage and discipline relationship. The slave always trusts that the Master will never genuinely hurt her. The slave gives her Master permission to whip or paddle or spank. That's not what I saw with Alex and Terry. She was truly afraid of her husband. Had he knocked out some of her teeth? I couldn't wait to get out of there.

To my surprise, out in the parking lot William offered my services to Alex. I'm sure William knew of my disgust because I kept shooting him meaningful glances. But there in the empty parking lot William had me kneel and kiss Alex's feet. What's more, he suggested I give Alex a blow job in the back of his van. I almost fainted. How could William do that to me? Luckily Alex declined my Master's generous offer. "We have to get home to the kids," Alex stammered.

William chuckled all the way home. He couldn't believe that Alex had refused a treat from his beautiful slave. But I was fuming.

"How could you offer me to someone I clearly didn't like?"

Again, my Master laughed at my foolishness. "That's part of being a slave. You don't always get what you want. Besides, I would have been right outside to protect you. It was just a test, Aileen. (Aileen was my "slave" name.) I wanted to see if you were willing to please me."

Back at my apartment, William and I engaged in a verbal session. He talked while I played with my pussy. Then I was commanded to get on my knees and worship my Master's cock with my mouth. William took a long time to reach a climax, prolonging it, holding back to make my chore that much more difficult. When he was ready to shoot, he had me lie down on the floor naked. Showering me with his jism, William made me lie there as it dried to a white crust on my skin. He called me his "cum receptacle." I was not permitted to wash and had to stay there for a full half-hour after he left. Perhaps I was a bad slave, because I stayed supine for only five minutes before I got up, laughing at my own foolishness, and jumped into the shower.

My senses dulled by the warm steam, I had to admit that I was quickly becoming bored with William. Perhaps it was because the sex was lacking in our relationship. It wasn't unpleasant acting out bizarre fantasies at his house, but I wanted more. William and I were on two different levels. He took the scene much too seriously. I wanted a lover and a companion to go out on the town with. I'd found a man to spank me, but he couldn't fuck me the way I desired or provide the passion I craved.

I found part of the submissive scene very attractive. Since it was so difficult for me to say "No" to anyone, it was very convenient to respond instead, "I'll have to ask permission from my Master." It was a way out, an excuse. But William was worming his way into things I felt didn't concern him. Cathy and I weren't allowed to swear in front of him. We couldn't even say "Yeah." It was always "Yes," preferably, "Yes, Master." When Cathy broke one of these rules, William forced her to bite down into a bar of Ivory soap. She complained endlessly about the nasty taste. The soap bore her teeth marks, a constant reminder of her punishment. William made her carry it around in her purse.

Cathy kept popping in and out of our lives. The focus kept switching. Sometimes she'd be more intensely involved with William than I was. At other times, I'd be his star slave. After a long absence, Cathy suddenly showed up on William's doorstep wearing a flowing white cotton dress and carrying a bunch of flowers. I was elated to see her. In a good mood because she had some cocaine with her, Cathy was at her best. William gave us permission to snort some coke. It was a drug that made me even more submissive. I felt freer and less inhibited when the powder was tingling in my nostrils. On that particular day, it was almost as though a curtain stood between me and reality. It created an illusion of love. I imagined that Cathy, William, and myself were one big, happy family. Well, maybe "The Addams Family" gone leather.

Our Master's next command was that we both assume the frisk position. We had stripped down to our bare skin and stood side by side with our arms above our heads. William was just introducing us to the whip at this time and he wanted Cathy to do the honors. She refused. "I can't hit her," Cathy explained, whip dangling in her fist. She and William argued mildly back and forth. There I was, legs stretched apart, arms starting to get numb as I held them above my head. I must have stood like that for thirty minutes as they talked. My body began to tremble and my muscles were giving out. Finally, I blurted out, "Just do it!" I actually started begging for it. My little performance was arousing our Master tremendously. When it was my turn to apply the whip to Cathy, I had no trouble at all since she had gotten me angry by making me wait so long for my own flogging. We used the whip lightly. It was more for show and stimulation than for inflicting actual pain. William was very pleased with our performance. To my surprise, I discovered that I enjoyed being dominant too, but I dared not tell my Master. I filed it away for a later date.

After the whipping, William had me do something I'd never done before. "Eat Cathy's pussy," he commanded with a glint in his eye. Now, he knew I didn't enjoy sexual contact with women, so perhaps that's why he made this request. Although Cathy and I had been in threesomes together, I had never performed this act on her. I was apprehensive. Cathy asked William not to force me to do something I didn't want to do. But William knew exactly what to say to sway her to his mode of thinking. "Don't you want a virgin, Cathy?" he teased.

As Cathy spread her legs apart, I looked for excuses. "I don't know how," I whispered.

Cathy pushed my hair back from my worried face. "Just do to me what you like done to yourself," she told me.

I did. At least, I tried. Cathy groaned with pleasure the moment my tongue sought out her clit. I was glad to give pleasure to my friend and also surprised that I wasn't repulsed by the act. So many men complain about the smell and taste of a cunt. I didn't find the pungent, charcoal-like taste very unpleasant. I wasn't aroused by lapping Cathy's pussy, but it was far more pleasant than tonguing my Master's asshole, something William had me do as part of my training. "I am a good slave," I kept telling myself as my friend's juices drenched my face. "I do whatever my Master tells me."

Halloween was a night Cathy and I were looking forward to. Dressed in our sluttiest gear, we expected William to take us to every kinky place in Hollywood. We told him to get dressed up too, but William still looked like a "fucking accountant," as Cathy liked to phrase it. Driving down Hollywood Boulevard, William got all bent out of shape when Cathy lit up a joint without asking his permission. Our evening of sleazy bar-hopping was cut short. William made a wild U-turn and headed back to his house. Cathy and I were about to be severely punished for our disrespect. Cathy and I were angry, but didn't say anything at first. We were all geared up for an evening on the town. William didn't know when to stop. He never stopped playing Master, overstepping the fine line between fantasy and reality. William tied Cathy up that night, and she started to complain. She wasn't in the mood, but he wouldn't understand.

Cathy's original enthusiasm held me back in my quest to be my Master's number one slave. I was envious of the fact that Cathy kept wearing William's collar. It was made of thick, brown leather, much like a dog's collar. She was ordered to wear it around her neck at home, to bed, and in places where it wasn't too conspicuous—to the supermarket, for example, but not to a family event. Cathy easily surrendered her mind and her body to William. I tried, but it was difficult because I was constantly analyzing the saneness of the entire situation. Perhaps this was my dominant tendency surfacing once more. Still, I craved to be the best, even if that meant being the best submissive. For now, anyway.

After the experience Halloween night, Cathy drifted out of our lives once more. This gave me another chance to become William's prize pupil. As we became more involved, he told me that soon I'd be ready to take my slave oath, which symbolized my devotion to him. Then I would be given the honor of wearing his collar. Perhaps the commitment frightened me. It was almost like becoming engaged and taking marriage vows in a standard type of relationship. Confused, I cut myself off from my Master. For weeks, I didn't phone him at my designated time. Although I loved being spanked, the rest of the submissive stuff grated against my sensibilities. I liked men, but the thought of getting down on my knees and worshipping them seemed odd. Why couldn't they get down on their knees and worship me once in a while? Intellectually I believed that both sexes were equal and one human being was not better than the other. For weeks, I severed myself from the scene.

This wasn't difficult, because I was immersed in studying for my licensing exams. It wasn't merely a written test. The second half involved standing before a board and discussing a case. The oral exam terrified me. Cathy was sweet enough to accompany me and wait until I was through. After the grueling tests were done, Cathy and I were up for excitement. Although we were always welcome at William's place, spending that night with him would have been too typical, too boring. We opted for a threesome with Sal, the dancer at the Queen Mary, but it didn't turn out to be very exciting. After he left, we were aching for more. Drunk and stoned, Cathy started calling ads in the *Free Press*.

A gentleman who offered spanking and Greek sounded interesting. He turned out to be a huge weightlifter who lived in West Los Angeles. Even though it was two in the morning, he invited us to his place. As soon as we arrived he grabbed me and put me over his knee to punish me for phoning so late. I really liked the way he pulled up my skirt and smacked his strong, firm hand against my ass. Soon we were tangled in a three-way in his bedroom. He kept taking breaks and dragging one of us into the living room for a royal spanking over his piano bench. It was arousing, but frenetic at the same time. He never talked very much. We didn't even know his real name. Finally, after a few hours, Cathy and I left with our buns tingling pink. We would often laugh about that evening, but never breathed a word about our encounter with "Baby Huey" to Master William.

Shortly thereafter, Cathy disappeared again. For lack of anything better, I called William. He was always willing to take me back. William was still the only person who could fulfill my spanking fantasy, but nevertheless our relationship once more became monotonous. A steady diet of spanking, dog training, and mutual masturbation can soon become boring.

The last night I saw William was Christmas Eve. It was a cozy evening filled with warm feelings. He gave me a beautiful gold ankle bracelet with the word "Slave" engraved on its surface. This made me feel sexy and positively slutty. It was license to unleash the sensuality I had repressed most of my life. I had also earned a thin, black, leather slave collar I enjoyed wearing to workout sessions and to the supermarket. I wondered if anyone realized what it meant. These accouterments made me feel like a member of a secret sexual organization, which, of course, I was. William also gave me a chain and a dog tag. I very brazenly had the gold tag engraved at a store in a suburban area. "Slave Aileen, Property of Sir William," it said. On the back, William instructed me to have engraved, "Total Whore." It was further proof to myself that I was "coming out of the closet."

That winter I treated myself to a Club Med vacation at Playa Blanca in Mexico. I figured it might soften the trauma of another Christmas alone. In those days, it was customary to share rooms. Vacationers usually picked their roommates on the plane trip down. One older man kept trying to convince me to bunk with his daughter, but I politely begged off. My attentions were directed toward a very tall, handsome, and blonde psychologist from San Diego. We began celebrating early when I joined the "Mile High Club" by treating him to a blow job in the bathroom. Once we got back to our seats, he informed me that he didn't want to restrict his activities to me at the club. That was fine with me.

Club Med was very much like TV's "Fantasy Island." We were greeted with cool, tropical drinks by the staff of good-looking men and women. One of their responsibilities was to be "sociable" with the opposite sex. I saw those guys as very fuckable love toys, much like the male dancers at the Queen Mary back home.

That night I was with my new-found San Diego friend. I suggested a three-way with his roommate, explaining that I was a sex slave and therefore programmed for pleasure. The word must have spread through the resort quickly because I wound up fucking and sucking tirelessly throughout the week, feeling like the perfect erotic servant. It felt very natural for me to share my charms with every man who desired them. Although Club Med resorts are known for their wildness, I must admit that my behavior shocked many of the other vacationers.

After three days, I wearied of the whole scene. I was drawn to Mr. San Diego, but he kept trying to ignore me. A few days later I attended a tropical picnic with a bunch of others. The moment we disembarked the bus, liquor was practically forced down our throats. In a remote, grassy meadow we played relay races and all sorts of silly games. We spun around and drunk rum as we spun. Very soon everyone was happily plastered. After lunch we were hot and ready for a swim in the Pacific. Suddenly a woman stripped off her bikini top and shouted to all of us, "Hey, look at my pierced nipples!" It was S&M, right at Club Med. Although I'd heard a lot about piercing, I'd never actually seen anyone display golden nipple rings in real life. I was more shocked to discover that this woman was Liza, the very same girl whose dad wanted me to room with his daughter. Assuming she was a prude, I turned down his offer and was stuck sharing my lodgings with a stuffy librarian from Arizona. On the bus ride back to our rooms, I managed to sit next to her. After a few moments of conversation, Liza asked me, "Are you a slut slave, too?" Very involved in S&M and very open about it, Liza and I became fast friends. Unlike me, Liza had a Master whom she was sexually attracted to *and* loved. Some slaves had everything! After that, Liza and I wreaked havoc wherever we went. We hooked up with a set of twenty-one-year-old twins from Long Island and their cute brother. We were hell on wheels. Since Liza was bi, we often indulged in threesomes, even orgies. Half the time it was such a tangle of arms and legs I wasn't sure who was doing what to me. Two of the guys were identical twins and that confused matters even further.

It was wonderful having a woman to discuss the S&M scene with. Liza opened me up to a whole new philosophy—S&M as fun! An upper-class, intellectual version of Cathy, Liza introduced me to a series of fantasy books about events in a place called "Gor." In one book, the females were dominant Mistresseses. In another, they were all submissive slaves. Liza and her Master's trip was taking to heart the whole Gorian trip. She liked to dress up sexily and serve him food. Liza enjoyed the lighthearted side of S&M. Her Master was her boyfriend and she had absolutely no fear of him. When we got back to L.A., Liza promised to introduce us. There was also another place she knew I'd like, "Peanuts," a lesbian bar that also featured drag queen shows.

Back at home, I avoided calling William. What was the point? I craved a Master who would also be my passionate lover, something he just couldn't be. But time and loneliness won out, as it usually did. I broke down and phoned William. He was glad to hear from me, as usual. He was especially thrilled to learn of my alliance with Liza. We soon made arrangements to meet with Liza and her Master, Paul. Since she and Paul were about seven years younger than me, there was a big age gap between them and William, who was well into his forties. We managed to have an enjoyable encounter despite those differences. Instead of playing together, I became Paul's slave while William plied his dog trip on Liza. I found Paul adorable and very fuckable. There was a bit of spanking before Paul settled down to eat my pussy. It was an act that I enjoyed immensely. It was so long since I'd had a delicious, inquisitive tongue exploring the folds of my vulva, and Paul seemed to savor every lick. Of course, William commented later on that Paul wasn't a "real" Master. Why? Because he was fun and loving? The rift between William and I grew when I saw what else was available.

Although we didn't have another four-way scene after that, Liza introduced me to another sensual treat. She took me to my first Janus meeting. The Janus Society is composed of people wholeheartedly involved in hedonistic lifestyles. They engage in pleasures of all varieties, from S&M to cross-dressing to anything else. I was anxious to be amid the free, "anything goes" atmosphere. My hopes were shattered as soon as I walked into the room. The average age seemed to be an older, withered-looking fifty-five. The few who were my age seemed dirty and scroungy. No one even came close to my standard gauge of "stripper cute."

In another way, however, there was more than I'd ever dreamed of. A black woman was strapped down to a piece of bondage tableware. I'd never seen anything like that before and it was a bit upsetting, reminding me of a scene from *Mandingo*. The meeting's program concerned body piercing—Liza's favorite subject. Nipple rings, body ornaments, tattoos, and play piercing was to Liza what spanking was to me. Today, Liza has ten holes in her ears, a pierced labia, a pierced clitoris, and a recently pierced tongue. She's also intrigued by tattooing. Her arms and her entire back are covered with intricate, winglike designs. Although our fetishes are decidedly different, Liza and I are still good friends.

Wine was served at the Janus meeting, so, as usual, I had more than my fill. When they needed a volunteer for a nipple-piercing demonstration, Liza prodded me to be the guinea pig. However, even in my drunken state, my sanity crept in. After the program, I was somehow grabbed by a bunch of people and found myself on the bondage table, but the owner of the house quickly scattered us. He hadn't given "permission" for us to use his dungeon. I still managed to find myself sprawled over an array of laps receiving spankings from men and a number of women. I thoroughly enjoyed it, but, in my inebriated state, couldn't help but wonder how I got there.

The week I'd spent at Club Med refueled my love of going out nights and partying. I grew more determined than ever to find a way to make a living through more pleasant channels, not ruling out sex. I was fed up and frustrated. I was an officially licensed psychologist, but the struggle to succeed wasn't changing. I took more dead-end jobs to support myself.

Then, out of the blue, my opportunity knocked. I ran into Sam again, the first man I'd slept with after my split with Daniel. Sam now had a girlfriend named Connie. I was still so hotly in lust with him that I did a three-way with the both of them. I really wanted to just be with him, but half the time my head was between Connie's legs or vice versa. In those days, I'd do almost anything just to be with a guy I wanted. If I got myself really high on Quaaludes or wine, it really didn't matter. When your brain is obliterated, you'd be surprised at what you'll do.

After that experience, Connie and I became friendly. When she made plans to meet an acquaintance at the Chalet, she asked me to tag along. I'd confessed my curiosity about the place and she didn't want to go there alone. Afterward, we could meet Sam at the Queen Mary. William had often spoken about the Chalet, but he'd never taken me inside as he'd promised.

I had just started a terrible new job at a women's hospital doing abortion counseling. The worst feature of the job wasn't that it involved abortions, but that it wasn't really counseling. When women came in, I had to explain the procedure to them and hold their hand through everything. I learned to rattle off a canned speech, like a bored tour guide at Disneyland. There was no real counseling, no feeling of contribution or of making a mark. On top of that, my supervisor had a very condescending attitude toward me and I wasn't making any more money than I had before I'd gotten my license. I had to work on Saturdays from seven a.m. to three p.m. and it was cutting into my nocturnal recreational habits. And then a new door opened my life.

9

Chalet

The entrance to the Chalet was very dark. There was a distinct, musty, smoky odor. After we were buzzed in, a door opened up on a young man sitting behind a desk. This was Vinnie. Behind him a neon sign glowed on the wall announcing "The Chalet." All of the necessary S&M equipment was on display. Whips. Paddles. Riding crops. We went upstairs to the lounge where Connie's friend was seated. The lounge looked almost like a typical living room. A kitchen was set off to the side where a pot of coffee was brewing. About ten people were gathered around a huge television showing a bondage video. There was one very gaunt, elderly man present. I learned that he was Frank Campbell, an illustrious writer of leathersex stories. Compared to the others in the room, he looked fairly "normal."

The other inhabitants seemed as though they were dressed for a bizarre costume party. Perhaps they were. There was Val, with a long, spiked, punk-rocker hairdo. Lacquered in heavy makeup and sporting claws for fingernails, Val was the top Dominant on call for the evening. Tammy seemed to be in her mid-forties. She wore a blue silk slave's tunic. Mariko was a light-skinned black girl who passed for oriental. She had black, flowing hair and wore a body-hugging vampirette's dress. Tall, busty, brunette Sheila was adorned as a harem girl. Then there was Nina. She didn't seem to fit at all. Looking like a Barbie doll masquerading as a prostitute, she wore a black negligee. Finally, Connie saw her friend. She'd been hooking for him and was meeting him to pick up some money. He, in turn, was there because he enjoyed tying women up.

Everyone seemed friendly enough and Nina even offered to take us on a tour. There was something about her warm manner that I liked. As we walked down the corridor, Nina revealed that she had previously been a nursery school teacher. The money available at the Chalet became too tempting, so she left her career in education. Here, the women earned about fifty dollars an hour, depending on the customer's fantasy. This didn't even include tips. The night before, Nina had picked up four hundred dollars in just a few hours. She was sure that I could earn that too. Silently agreeing with her, I knew I was more authentic than Nina was. I wouldn't be doing it just for the money. William had trained me well as a slave and I was sure I could bring others pleasure. I had a marketable skill, so to speak. I knew I could take an intense spanking or flogging if necessary. I was very good at it. Most of the girls at the Chalet weren't truly into S&M. They were just play-acting for the money. In contrast, I was living the life of a submissive for free.

Each room had a certain flavor. Painted a pretty aqua blue, the Queen's Room was inspired by *The Story of O.* There were two whipping posts from which slaves could be strung up and thrashed. It was even equipped with a Catherine Wheel, named after a saint who'd been tortured. The victim was bound to a crosslike structure and spun around. This was Nina's favorite object in the whole place. With her eyes bright, she described how wonderful it felt to be tied down to it, helpless. Downstairs was the Spanish Room. Very large, its walls and floors were covered with tiles. It contained a suspension bar. This made it possible to hang someone from the ceiling. There was also a stock, a pillory, and a cage for further imprisonment. The Black and White Room was named in honor of a famous bondage photographer. Inside there was a suspension bar and little else. Upstairs was the Hank Lipton Room. When I became a working girl at the Chalet, it would become my favorite because it was smaller, more atmospheric than the Spanish Room. In addition to the customary suspension bar, there was a soft, cushioned bondage table suitable for tying people down upon. I noticed that the hooks were well within reach, even for someone as tiny as I was. It was a very manageable, almost cozy room, if a dungeon could be considered cozy.

After the tour, Nina took me for an audience with the Master of the house, Sir Kevin. His private office was called the "Headquarters." Starry-eyed, I walked into a fantasy. As I waited for Sir Kevin to respond to my feeble knock on his door, I wondered if I should fall onto my knees and crawl into the inner sanctum. Laughing at myself, I thought better of it and entered timidly. In his late fifties, Sir Kevin cut a striking figure. I was immediately intimidated by his tall, lean, bearded form. Despite his forboding looks, Kevin was surprisingly easy to talk to and had a kindly air about him. I explained that I was a real slave.

"Trouble with your Master," he concluded knowingly.

"Not exactly," I began, explaining that William and I were growing apart.

As you must have concluded by now, *The Story of O* is something of a yardstick to which many aspects of S&M are compared. To better understand what I was looking for, Sir Kevin wondered aloud whether I was more attracted to the younger Master in the story, named Renee, or the older man, Sir Stephan. Without a moment's hesitation, I chirped, "Renee." Being an older gentleman himself, I could see Kevin's mild disappointment, but he suggested that I take a closer look at Vinnie, the handsome gentleman at the front desk. He had just completed his Master training and was looking for an obedient, attractive female slave. Somehow, I summoned up the courage to ask Sir Kevin for a job at the Chalet. "I'm sure we could find a place for you," he said without a moment's hesitation. I thought it would be more difficult securing this kind of employment. I thought there might be an audition or a trial run. But no, Sir Kevin seemed confident that I would do well at his establishment. I felt flattered at his decision. I had never considered myself overly attractive. It was the first time I'd been hired for my looks. In truth, I was flattered and frightened. Could I really do this? Would men really pay dearly for the privilege of dominating me? I informed Sir Kevin that I had another career that I prefered be kept a secret.

"Are you a member of the CIA?" he inquired, half-jokingly.

"A therapist," I admitted.

Kevin was sure that my background could only help me in my work at the Chalet. In addition to the commercial business of fantasy fulfillment explored at the Chalet, there was also a "church" dedicated to the S&M lifestyle. Kevin invited me to attend the next meeting of the "Order of Poses," which was legally recognized as a church for tax purposes. It had meetings on Sundays, to which all slaves were commanded to attend naked. He was sure I'd feel right at home with all of the other male and female submissives.

Although the prospect of working at the Chalet was very exciting and Kevin sensed I'd be a "natural," he suggested I come back to meet Kira, his partner in the operation. Since I was already feeling submissive toward this strong male character, I obeyed. Friday was my day off. Taking a deep breath, I walked into the Chalet again, thrilled to see that Vinnie was at the front desk again. Nina was there and delighted to see me. Immediately I felt at home, but soon discovered that five o'clock in the afternoon wasn't the best time to observe a typical day at the Chalet. I took advantage of the lull and spoke to Vinnie. He was many things that William wasn't, including very attractive. I imagined how his strong arms could thrill me, hurt me, and at the same time protect me. The only drawback was that he was already involved with someone. Oddly enough, it was a lady who wasn't intrigued by the S&M scene.

Since I had to see a private therapy client, I had to leave, but made sure to rush back by ten that evening to see Kira. She was supposed to be arriving from Las Vegas. Although I wasn't certain why it was so vital that I meet her, I followed Sir Kevin's orders. I was very good at following orders. The crew was different at the Chalet at night. A man named Billy sat behind the desk. A former truck driver, he was missing his front teeth. He was an odd personality indeed, and called women "Sis." Billy made a big fuss when he saw me, but he was Kira's slave. This fact confused me because I knew that Kira was Kevin's slave. I didn't think a slave could have a slave, but at that point I had a lot to learn.

Kira was late. She arrived in a flurry that was customary for her. Wearing a fur coat, she had leashes attached to several yapping Pekinese dogs. Looking more like a queen than a slave, Kira was about five foot five with long, dark hair and huge breasts. There was something about her that immediately made me feel uncomfortable. She was very cold and distant. After Kira got herself settled, I was invited back to the Headquarters for a closed-door discussion. Obviously, I'd made quite an impression on Kevin, but it was clear that I had to get the approval of the queen bee before I was hired. Kevin valued the fact that I was a "true submissive," which, as William had told me, was a rare quality indeed. Suddenly all of my bad points, my weaknesses, were turned into positive things. Not liking to make decisions, not liking to be in control were the marks of a perfect submissive. Perhaps that is what set Kira off. When she discovered that I was a therapist, she made a point of stressing how much she helped the girls psychologically. Much of her slave training was focused on getting the girls off drugs. In fact, Kira kept emphasizing the fact that people at the Chalet didn't do drugs. Did she think I was an undercover narcotics officer? I would later learn that she was a heavy cocaine user. For some reason, Kira seemed hell-bent on impressing me.

I told Kevin and Kira that I was a submissive, but that there was one thing about it that bothered me. Could I be a slave *and* a feminist at the same time? It seemed to be a contradiction. Kevin informed me that Kira was a staunch feminist and he even "permitted" (another contradiction) her to attend NOW meetings. Kira saw nothing wrong with standing up for women's rights in society, yet at the same time allowing herself to be chained for hours, waiting naked on the floor for her Master's arrival.

Although I sensed Kira didn't like me, she admitted that I would do well as a working submissive. She even expressed an interest in taking me on as her private slave, an idea that didn't appeal to me in the least. I had my sights set on Vinnie. Why did the wrong people always want me as their slaves?

Kira assured me that everything was on the up and up at the Chalet. There was absolutely no sex between girls and clients. That was illegal. Just to get a taste of what really went on behind those secretive doors, she suggested I come back and observe a session the next afternoon. My virgin viewing experience was in the Spanish Room. It was usually illuminated with candlelight, which cast wonderful shadows on the tile-work. The session turned out to be much more intense than those that usually transpired within the confines of the Chalet. Velvet was the Dominatrix running the show. She was a tough old bitch who always reminded me of the sadistic guard who always turns up in those low-budget female prison movies, the one who takes great pleasure in tormenting a nubile inmate. A confirmed lesbian, Velvet was very sadistic in her dominance toward men. She claimed to have had a ranch in Oklahoma filled with male slaves. But I would later discover that most of the stories these ladies told were untrue. When you're paid to enact fantasies for other people, I suppose you have to have fantasies of your own.

Velvet didn't enjoy casual bondage, teasing, or sensuality. It was a double session. Mistress Allie, a sweet black lady, did the preliminaries.

That was "light" stuff: verbal humiliation, mild whippings. All the male customer requested was some teasing, but he also requested that Velvet pierce his cock. That's very much out of the norm. Very few clients request it.

I watched the action from a corner, naked and on my knees. I was content with fading into the background of this bizarre scene. Velvet and Mistress Allie told me what to do and included me in on the insanity. I was shocked when they actually put a long needle through the poor man's penis. Part of me wanted to cry out and run, but the other part was so intent on being a good slave that I remained glued to my spot on the ground. Blood was dripping onto the floor. The Mistresses ordered me to touch the man's penis, to hold it in my hand. I had to play with it. His blood coated my fist.

Despite this harrowing introduction, I agreed to start working at the Chalet the very next day. Slated for a split shift from four to midnight, the idea of having something definite to do on a Saturday night appealed to me. I bought a skimpy black teddy to wear for the occasion. At one o'clock that afternoon, my phone rang. It was Vinnie. "Sweetheart," he explained, "one of the girls didn't show up. Could you get here early? We need you."

We need you. Those words were music to my ears. It had been such a long time since I felt truly needed for anything. I had other plans, but changed them and rushed to get ready. "Just be here," Vinnie commanded. He informed me that he would give me a stroke of a riding crop on my ass for every minute I was late. Was that a promise, or a threat?

I arrived ten minutes past Vinnie's deadline, and I savored every stroke of punishment he gave me. Bending over his knee, I was elated. I was working and living out a fantasy besides. There was purpose to my life once again. I had friends at the Chalet. We were a little family of sadists and masochists. I was sure it would be more like a paid vacation than a job. At first I told myself that I would only work Friday and Saturday nights for a few weeks. But soon I became an addict to the attention, to the money. It became almost impossible to suffer through my dreadful day jobs and I soon quit them.

From this point on, my life gets very difficult to talk about. It's times like these when I really wish I had a close friend—someone who would sit here beside me, talking me through my conflicting emotions. Instead, I'm sitting here alone with a tape recorder. It's painful for me to remember how fragile I was emotionally when I began working at the Chalet. It's almost embarrassing. I was very lonely and felt as though everyone and everything had abandoned me. Suddenly I was wanted. Formerly a totally unnecessary object, I was now sought out. The Chalet gave some structure to my life, a purpose, somewhere to go.

I decided to take a new name. I wasn't William's slave Aileen anymore, and I certainly wasn't Alice. I christened myself "Jacqueline," partly after a character in *The Story of O,* and partly because I liked it. Jacqueline was a pretty name. Not like Alice. Alice was dowdy. Alice was scared. Alice was ugly. She reminded me too much of the past. I never wanted to be Alice again. From that moment on, I became Jacqueline. Nonetheless, Jacqueline felt a little dubious sitting around and waiting for customers with the odd menagerie at the Chalet. What was I doing here? But almost from the moment I arrived, I was a busy little slave. Perhaps the men who came in saw how committed I was to the scene.

Frank tied me up in the Queen's Room, where I was on display for all of the clients who walked by browsing. One after the other, customers came in to admire me. A handsome young man arrived and requested me for his session, nothing too complicated, just a bit of spanking and light bondage. I was so aroused that I ended up giving him a blow job, fully aware that it was against Chalet rules. Although some girls secretly used the premises to hook, that wasn't my intention. I really thought this guy was cute and wanted to have him inside me. I wasn't doing it for the money. Maybe I did it for the attention, or for an illusion of love. Sitting with him in the lounge afterward, I felt as though we were on an authentic date.

Before my next shift, Kira called me into the Headquarters. "Jacqueline," she snapped, "I heard you were fraternizing with one of the customers." Immediately I wondered which one of my jealous co-workers had ratted on me. Although Kira was visibly upset, she knew I wasn't a "working girl." I was much too innocent for that. I did receive a stern warning. "If we ever catch you doing anthing like that, we'll force you to wear a chastity belt. And *I'll* hold the key." Naturally, I believed Kira's every word. After all, complete trust was part of being a good slave. That was the only time I broke the club's celibacy rules.

It soon became clear that the other girls were envious of my success. I had so much energy that I was able to see one client after the other and I was certainly in demand. Each Friday I went to the bank to deposit a large wad of cash. Miraculously, my savings account began to grow. I felt very legitimate, a personification of the phrase, "Laughing all the way to the bank." I was doing that, literally, plus I was enjoying myself.

There were myriad sessions. It was a procession of faces. My days were booked solid. Jacqueline was busy, busy, busy, while the other girls sat in the lounge sullenly drinking coffee and watching the afternoon soaps. What they didn't understand was that I wasn't faking my enjoyment of the submissive's lifestyle, as they were. I was totally immersed in my work. I was trying my damndest to be "Miss Perfect," but I often felt as though I were a child at the Chalet. All of the Mistresses were mother figures to me. Kevin and Kira were sordid samples of parents. It was bizarre.

I still remember many of my early clients' trips. One guy would come in and watch me masturbate in front of a mirror. I'd go absolutely crazy, giving him his full money's worth, talking the way William had taught me. Another customer came in with a bunch of old clothes he'd collected from thrift shops. He'd make his girls put them on, and we'd go through a spanking scenario. One of his favorite story lines had me billed as a naughty secretary. I had the choice of either getting fired or getting spanked for messing up an important job. Of course, I opted to get my fanny swatted. Wearing a long skirt and bulky sweater, he'd hike up my dress and hit me soundly as I lay across his knees. My first double session was with Mistress Val. She played a schoolteacher to my naughty student. In this tale, the teacher discovered the client and me playing with each other's genitals in class. To his great delight, both he and I were soundly punished. Another client wanted me to call myself "Cunt." He'd bring me a pair of panties and then tear them off my body. In addition, he liked to tie me up in all sorts of odd positions. I was really very patient back then and put up with things I'd never consider doing today. Behind it all was my quest for acceptance. I was wanted. I was providing a service that people needed.

Gil used to come to the Chalet late at night. He kept telling me that he wanted a "golden shower" (urinating on his body), yet always tried to fight it. He'd be so stoned that I'd literally have to chase him around the room. "Oh, Mistress, I want you to piss on me." He'd further embellish his desire with a detailed story. "I'm in Las Vegas with you," Gil would say. "We're in the restaurant of a beautiful hotel. You have to go to the bathroom very badly, but you wouldn't have to get up—

I could be your toilet." Then Gil would pant and position his head as though he really were a toilet. Deep down, I don't think he really wanted me to urinate on him. It was just the thought, the idea that I might, that aroused him so fully. Besides that, "golden showers" were also against Chalet rules. One night, though, Gil convinced me to go through with it. At first I couldn't bring myself to do it, but somehow I managed to dribble a bit of urine onto his face. As soon as I did, he freaked out and left.

Like clockwork, every Friday night for two or three years, Jim Smith booked a session with me. He requested the same thing every time. We'd go into the Queen's Victorian Room and he'd arrange two chairs facing each other in opposite corners of the room. Then he'd bring in some magazines from the lounge. For a half hour or so, we'd sit there reading, not even looking at each other.

Suddenly, he'd say, "Excuse me, where's the bathroom?"

"Down the hall and to your left," I'd answer.

It took me a few months to finally realize what Jim was doing. During his bathroom breaks, he'd snort cocaine. When he returned, we'd resume our reading. All Jim wanted me to do was subtly tease him. The first time, I brazenly spread my legs wide open. "No, no," he cried. That's not what he wanted. I had to spread them apart just an inch at a time. Very slowly, over the course of the hour. I also had to wear the same long, black dress in every session. "Excuse me, do you know the time?" he'd ask next. Or perhaps it was, "Could you watch my things while I go to the bathroom?" At this point, his time was often up. Sometimes, he'd choose to stay for another half hour to engage in more silly conversation. Other times, Jim and I were supposed to be students meeting for the first time in the campus library. He was very specific about the facts. I was a senior and he was a sophomore. We had the same psychology teacher and would talk about his class, about the exams we were cramming for. Then he'd say his customary, "Excuse me, I have to go to the bathroom." When he came back, we'd talk some more. Sometimes we'd pretend that we had gone back to my room to study. Again, I would have to seduce him, opening my legs slightly, slowly, subtly. Sometimes, Jim would be shaking uncontrollably from all of the cocaine that was zooming through his system. We'd make believe the phone would ring. I'd answer it, talking to an imaginary friend. "Yeah, Suzie," I'd say to no one in particular, "Jim's here. He's really cute. Oh sure, I'm going to fuck him. Right.

I'll call you later and tell you all about it." At that point, Jim would inevitably do something that I'd have to berate him for. I'd make him take off his clothes (he always wore a pair of pink panties), tie him up lightly and spank him a bit, endlessly taunting him about his panties. When the buzzer rang, signifying that our session was over, he'd cry, "That's it?" and leave. He never climaxed.

Interestingly enough, I ran into Jim at a drug rehab meeting a few years ago. I was very glad to see that he was sober, but the funny thing was that he could barely remember my name or any of the things we'd done together. Only after I reminded him did he laugh and admit that I was a big part of his "Fourth Step." That's a term in the group for the time when you let out your secrets and share them with someone. Jim and I met a few times at meetings, but when we tried to do a session sober it didn't work out.

Another client that sticks in my memories is a huge man named Nick. He used to visit often and usually did a session with Mistress Kim and me for three or four hours. Nick requested that I parade around wearing shackles on my legs.

"Who are you?" Nick would bellow.

"Number 05748930" I'd respond.

Wild-eyed, Nick often brandished a knife. He could get very crazy and out of control. That's why Kim was there, to keep him in check. Toward the very end of the session, Nick would recite Kaddish, a very sacred Jewish prayer for the dead. I never understood why he did this. But there was some sweetness to the man. Nick gave me a copy of the book *9½ Weeks*. He also liked to call me his *shayna maidel,* which means "pretty girl" in Yiddish.

Day after day, I felt as though I were an actress cast into unusual roles in an avant-garde theater. I portrayed different characters throughout the night. Jerry was into spanking, so we got along famously. I was his naughty niece in dire need of a thrashing to set her straight. Jerry knew how to get into the verbal aspects of spanking as well. At one point it began to seem like "The Perils of Jacqueline," a continuing saga that went on three or four times a week. Jerry would refer to previous sessions and I struggled to remember the intricate details of our game.

There was another man who used to supply his own outfits. He was a harmless type who also liked to tie girls up, and we were all very sad to learn that he killed himself a few years after he stopped visiting the Chalet. Perhaps, without an outlet, he couldn't deal with his bottled-up fantasies.

There was another suicide by a former customer, Tony, but I don't think there is any relationship between visiting S&M parlors and suicide. If anything, indulging in a place like the Chalet is a release mechanism that allows people to live out fantasies and then carry on normal lives. Tony liked to try to figure out what other people's trips were. Like an emotional chameleon, he would adjust himself to whatever turned you on. Since I enjoyed being a submissive, he'd stroke his cock as he talked about a waitress he knew. "Annie had a big, old, fat ass," he'd say. "Viv, the restaurant manager, asked me what I could do to straighten her out since Annie had been bad lately. So, I'd bend Annie over the table and fuck her in the ass." Tony's story was endless. I'd usually help him embellish the story, or else egg him on, feigning interest and asking questions. "And then what did you do, Tony?" It was basically a talking session during which Tony harmlessly masturbated himself to a climax. Years later, he blew his brains out.

The clients I saw during my early days at the Chalet were very different from the ones I have today. It's pretty standard now. I'm the Mistress, the one in control. In those days, though, I did whatever was requested of me. Spanking was probably the most common request. I would take it hour after hour. Paddlings. Whippings. Men would tie me up in various ways. Often I shared the scene with other Mistresses. They'd protect me if a client became too intense. During one frightening incident, both a Mistress and her customer tried to dominate me at the same time. They dripped hot candlewax on my skin, but they didn't hold the candle up high enough, so the wax burned me.

Although we were rarely on the same shifts together, Nina and I were becoming very close. We were both tiny, with long blonde hair, and I suppose Kevin wanted to give the clients some variety. A client once chose both Nina and me to work as a team. He wanted me to dominate Nina. A diehard submissive, I didn't really know what I was doing. I strapped my friend to the extension bar, hoisting her up without looking. Suddenly, she was dangling off the floor squealing, "Jacqueline, let me down!" Our client wondered aloud if he'd booked a session with Tweedledee and Tweedledum.

An old Jewish man named Irwin was also a frequent visitor. Today there are only two clubs still open in Los Angeles, but in those days there were probably about seven. Irwin hopped from club to club, looking for new girls to try out. Every day he would call and ask if there were any new girls available. A handful of other customers were also interested in breaking in nubile submissives. Vinnie warned me that Irwin was "heavy," but that didn't faze me. I was "Super Slave," and I wanted to impress Vinnie with the amount of punishment I could take.

Alone together in the room, Irwin told me, "I speak little. You speak less." He took his scene very seriously, but I just couldn't. He had this comical little Jewish accent and I couldn't help laughing. I suggested we bring Nina in on the session. When she saw me with my wrists and ankles bound and at the mercy of this silly gnome, she burst out laughing too. Irwin was so angry that he chased me around the room with a whip. Even though he was slow, I couldn't get away because I was still shackled. He beat me with such a fury that it left marks on my body. We ended the session immediately.

I met Dale when I was still a beginner at the Chalet. He immediately whipped out his enrollment card to convince me that he was a charter member of the club. Supposedly that meant I could do more with him than with anyone else. Dale began with a basic session, followed by something he called the "extra special session." A basic session consisted of kissing his feet. The "extra" garnered a big tip and concluded with a blow job. The girls at the Chalet had a type of rating system when a new girl started—was she the sort of girl who'd give Dale head? I wasn't.

Other, more exotic clients were Tom Bondage and Hardware Rick. Rick's trip was really strange. Generally, he'd want a female Dominant, but sometimes he'd take a submissive. He was very into stomachs and loved watching a woman's belly ripple. With a submissive like me, he'd tie her down tight and press a vibrator against her clit. There was nothing erotic or sexy about it. The intensity was almost painful, but Rick enjoyed watching her stomach flutter as she climaxed violently. Rick did have an excellent piece of equipment—Hitachi's Magic Wand. It's easily the best vibrator on the market, but his technique was very harsh. When it was Rick's turn to be submissive, he wanted to be tied down tightly and serviced by two Mistresses. One would have to punch his stomach very hard while the other held a heavy-duty vibrator against his dick. We dubbed him "Hardware Rick" because he carried all of these odd devices with him. One gadget actually pumped up his stomach. Then you'd have to actually punch the air out of it. We had a theory that Rick possessed a secret pregnancy fantasy and that he was trying to simulate the condition. He was a very educated man with a doctorate in physics. He assured us that he'd consulted a doctor who told him that his stomach technique wasn't harmful. Despite his supposed intelligence, however, Hardware Rick was a very sad case. He often talked about how normal sex didn't turn him on anymore. He was another S&M club hopper, going from club to club pursuing his fantasy.

Another odd customer was a man who liked to spank us not on, but between the cheeks of our asses. The gross part about it was that he'd want us to spank him in the same spot. He had such terrible hemorrhoids that by the time you finished spanking him he'd be almost bloody. Back in those days, I didn't know where to draw the line. I thought I was supposed to take anything a customer dished out. One time a man with a heavy southern accent spanked me until I was almost sobbing. The next week, he thrashed Nina. She was angry with me because I hadn't warned her about how brutal he had been, but to me it was nothing. I thought I was doing just what I was supposed to do.

During those early days at the Chalet, I was determined to impress Vinnie. We only worked together on Tuesday nights, but he was my savior behind the desk. Since we were fully computerized, one of his chores was to log on all of the sessions the girls did. It became very important to me that he be aware of my popularity. Somehow I thought it would please him. He would see in black and white what a good, sought-after submissive I was. Every time I was in a session I would think about Vinnie. I kept hoping that soon I'd be doing these things with him. It wasn't all one-sided. Often he'd wonder aloud why he was living with his girlfriend, Lila, instead of me. He asked me pointed questions about how I'd treat him in certain situations. In short, he was leading me on and I was falling for him.

One night, Vinnie finally took me out. Because Lila was at their apartment, we went to his parents' home. When we crawled into the bed he'd slept in as a little boy, it felt so good. We didn't make love or anything, just held each other. I felt very cradled, very protected just lying beside him. In a soft voice, Vinnie explained that he needed a month or so to break up with Lila. He wanted to let her down easy, and I thought that was admirable of him. When he was finally free of her, things would blossom with us. That was his promise. A month seemed like a reasonable amount of time, so I waited patiently for Vinnie, and as I waited I devoted myself to becoming a star submissive, hoping he would notice.

Once a month the Chalet featured special shows. I believe Kevin charged guests fifty dollars to attend, and would often have the gall to serve them Kentucky Fried Chicken for that high price. But the food wasn't the major draw of the Chalet exhibitions. My first one was a Valentine's Day pageant. Each of us girls served a different purpose that night. One was completely covered in chocolate cake icing. Nina was a Kewpie doll. I walked out naked, wearing nothing but edible body paint. Wandering around the room, I urged everyone present to lick me. Being an exhibitionist, I was ecstatic. There was no shame or embarrassment. I was proud to be a submissive.

That night, the biggest scene took place downstairs. I was a little frightened when I walked into the Spanish Room. There was Billy, all strung up. Kira was giving him a full-blown flogging. There was nothing playful about it. I was haunted by overtones of the way slaves were actually tortured in the Deep South. It disgusted me to watch Billy squirming and jerking. The oddest thing was that afterward Billy was smiling and telling everyone how much he enjoyed it.

When I approached Kira about the extreme violence, she explained that Billy sometimes needed scenes like that. She made it sound almost therapeutic, telling me that she often whipped him hard to "vent" him. It turned out that Billy really did look forward to those horrible beatings. If any length of time went by and they neglected to flog him, Billy would be walking around almost in tears. "I need to get whipped," he'd sob. "Mistress doesn't even whip me anymore!" When Kira finally relented, he'd be calm and grinning his toothless grin for days. I've also experienced that kind of euphoria after very intense scenes. You feel a sense of calm and relief when it's over. When you're focusing in on the feelings and you're screaming, you have no choice but to let every ounce of tension out of your body. But today I can't help but think that the hard trips are too severe, no matter how tranquil you feel later on.

After that party I teased Kevin and sarcastically told him it had been a pretty tame evening, explaining that he should offer something more authentic the next time. In the back of my mind, I was hoping I could do a dramatic public scene with Vinnie and finally prove to him what an excellent slave I was. Kevin just gave me a strange look and said, "We'll see."

At one of my early sessions a very attractive client requested foot worship. It wasn't too difficult for me to sit on his chest and let him kiss and worship my toes and run his tongue between them. Naive as I was back then, I just couldn't believe a man like him would come to the Chalet for something as simple as kissing a woman's feet. I thought it should have been easy enough for a man to get that kind of thing from his spouse or lover—unlike spanking, with its S&M overtones. Surely he shouldn't have to pay for it. I told Kevin that this customer could probably find someone like me in a bar. "No, he couldn't," Kevin informed me. "You're not in a bar. You're here."

The next month, the Chalet had another theme party. March brought the St. Patrick's Day Show. From the local erotic bakery came a huge, custom-made leprechaun with a hard-on. My job was to crawl out naked and eat the frosted prick to entertain the crowd. It really turned me on, even though I was performing for a crowd of horny old men.

After that little skit, Kevin finally invited me to come up and help him do something a bit more "real." I was expecting him to tie me up and whip me, honored that my boss had selected me out of all the other girls. Actually, I would have much preferred to be flogged by Vinnie, but at least he'd be watching. What I didn't know was that Kevin had chosen to punish me for my flippant comment after the first show. There was a weird aura in the Queen's Room as Kevin had a couple of women prepare me. They took off all my clothes and bound me very tightly to the columns. It was a scene right out of *The Story of O.* I wasn't very happy when they gagged and blindfolded me. There was dead silence. I was left alone in that room for quite a while. Suddenly I heard people filing in through the doorway. I heard Kevin announce to the spectators, "Jacqueline is very much aroused. Her cunt is probably wet and dripping." Sure enough, I was excited at the prospect of being shown off, though not particularly sexually aroused. I just played along.

I didn't know that before the guests were ushered into the Queen's Room, Kevin had told them that he was going to demonstrate how to "break" a slave. The customary way was to methodically whip the victim on strategic areas of the body, directly underneath the armpits, on the backs of the thighs. Not hard, just steadily, relentlessly. Kevin detailed the stages that a woman goes through just before she's fully broken. At first, she's very aroused. Then it becomes painful. Then she gets angry. But finally she submits. That's exactly what Kevin intended to do to me. At this point, I'm sure Kevin and Kira were hoping to make me their personal slave. They had done this with other girls. When Sue had a fight with her boyfriend/Master, they "broke" her and made her sign some sort of slave contract. Whenever Sue worried about some trivial problem, Kevin coolly told her, "You're my slave now. I'll take care of everything. You don't have to worry about anything anymore." To me, it was a comforting thought. I wanted to be a slave again, but older men like Kevin didn't attract me and neither did a woman like Kira. I didn't want to be a child again with nasty parents. I wanted a lover/Master—Vinnie.

I wanted Vinnie, but I wasn't going to get him that night. In the Queen's Room, Kevin took a very thick crop and began whipping me. He didn't concentrate too much under my arms, but kept snapping it against my thighs. He went back and forth, back and forth with the whip. At first it didn't hurt much, but after constant, steady pressure, the pain became almost unbearable. I kept praying that Kevin would stop, but he didn't. He was determined to get me to break down, although I didn't realize it at the time. I tried to take the beating, jerking about. But when I began screaming, Kevin took off my gag.

"Is there something you want to say?" he asked. "Have you had enough?"

I was very stubborn. "No," I told him angrily. Kevin shrugged and kept whipping me. The entire scene went on for about twenty minutes. Finally, I begged him to stop.

"If I stop, can I do anything to you?" Kevin asked.

I couldn't agree to that. I was afraid he'd claim me as his slave and coerce me to sign "slave papers." So I cried out, "No," over and over again. Kevin began whipping me again. Finally, the pain was too excruciating. I promised Kevin he could do anything he wanted if he'd just stop whipping me.

"Anything?" he asked wickedly.

"Yes," I told him.

"Well, then, I want to whip you some more," he said nastily.

Kevin eventually decided I'd had enough. The girls ran to get some ice to soothe my lashed body. It was a great relief to receive some tenderness. When I had the strength to go downstairs, I discovered that my thighs were terribly bruised and swollen. I was on the verge of tears, but at that moment Kira appeared. I wanted to fall into her arms and sob, but she stopped me. "No, Jacqueline," she said sternly. "There isn't time to cry. You're on duty tonight. Besides, you should be very proud of what you just did." Suddenly, I did feel very good. The other girls thought I was absolutely crazy to take such a violent beating, but Kira's praise swayed me. Immediately, even though I was hurting, I felt proud too. The next day, Kevin told me that there were only a handful of women in the United States who could endure a whipping to the extent that I had. Silently, I thought, "So what?" But another vulnerable part of me was convinced that I'd really accomplished something. Vinnie was on duty. I couldn't wait to show off my huge, round bruises to him. I thought he'd be impressed, of all people. But I could see from his shocked expression that he felt almost sorry for me. He didn't say a word.

The next show at the Chalet wasn't too heavy, but since it was held only two days before my birthday, I was in rare form. I was tied down and one of the clients put a candle deep into my vagina and lit the other end. The birthday girl was instructed to blow out the candle and make a wish. Afterward they soothed my glowing labia with ice. I still craved attention, and the big money I was earning made all sorts of atrocities acceptable.

Despite my various wild performances, I still wasn't able to seduce Vinnie. Sometimes he'd promise to phone me on my nights off, but he never did. Nonetheless, I was becoming emotionally attached to him. I created a fantasy and occasionally Vinnie would play along with me. I often wondered if Kevin had instructed Vinnie to humor me, only because Kevin didn't want to lose one of his biggest moneymakers—me. Whatever I made on a session, I split down the middle with Kevin. Every week my take-home pay was anywhere from seven hundred to eight hundred dollars. Kevin made the same, so I'm sure he didn't want to lose the income I brought in. Telling Vinnie to "keep Jacqueline happy" was a small consideration to ask of another worker.

Tab Parks (not his real name) was a big Hollywood producer who had presumably done Richard Pryor movies. He spent a lot of money during his sessions, but would never tip us girls. Kevin and Kira didn't care, just so long as the clients were paying the house. They always treated Tab nicely when he came calling, but none of the girls liked being with him. We submissives had a chamois whip that we liked out clients to use on us. It had a good sound, but very little bite. Although Tab would bring a chamois whip and a paddle into the room, he was usually interested in a talking session. I'd have to kneel at his feet as he described his beautiful mansion. "I'm going to buy you exquisite clothes, darling," he'd tell me. "Then I'm going to strip you naked and drag you outside. I'm going to whip every inch of your body. And darling, maybe if you're very good I'll give you to my dogs. You'd like that, wouldn't you? You'd like fucking a dog."

"Yes, Master," I'd pant. "I'd love fucking your dogs. It would be good for me." I would always enthusiastically murmur exactly what he wanted to hear.

Sometimes Tab would tell me that he was going to throw me into a jail cell full of unwashed prisoners.

"I'd want to see you suck off all of their big, fat crusty dicks, darling."

"Oh, yes," I'd moan. "Please give me those big, fat, crusty dicks. Oh, yes. . . ."

"It would be good for you darling," he'd say. "I know you like filthy cocks, darling."

But often, after only a few minutes, Tab would claim he was bored and simply walk out in the middle of a session. Another time Tab brought Vinnie in so that he could watch him whip me. It was the first time my dream Dominant had flogged me. It was pure bliss. A whip never felt so good. Vinnie was enacting my Master/slave fantasy. He owned me and I wanted to be able to accept any kind of pain for him. But outside of the Chalet, Vinnie always had some excuse about why he couldn't be with me. Either it was Lila's vulnerability because of her drinking problem or some other lame excuse. The months passed and there was still no Vinnie. I wanted him badly.

The Chalet was my entire life. I worked there steadily, five nights a week. Although some of the girls signed "slave papers" with Kevin and Kira, it was rare that their devotion lasted. Velvet brought her slave Esther to a party. Esther was ready to go through slave training and was very frightened of the prospect. Since she'd gone through basic training in the military she couldn't imagine it being much worse. Velvet was giving Esther over to Kevin and Kira for training. I later found out that "slave training" in their book consisted of going to their house in Las Vegas and taking care of Kira's son Sean, who was supposedly a terror. Slaves had to serve Kira breakfast in bed and do all the housework. To me, it didn't sound like "slave training," but getting free maid service. Someone told me about a former slave who, after serving Kira breakfast in bed, received total verbal humiliation because the tray wasn't set correctly. Kira threw the tray at her cowering slave and ordered that it be set again in the proper manner.

Kira's son Sean was about thirteen at that time. When he was almost eighteen, Sean started to work the Chalet's front desk. We became very friendly. Looking back at his bizarre adolescence, Sean told me how he hated many of the visitors to their Las Vegas home, especially Mistress Val. Val was commissioned to take care of Sean, which included picking him up from high school. Poor Sean was mortified because she looked so weird. She had long, black fingernails and was frequently at the house chilling out from snorting too much cocaine. I really liked Sean, but he was a child who grew into an adult with a lot of problems. Totally mother dominated, Sean is now gay.

One night Claire, a fellow worker at the Chalet, and I were on a shift together. I was all set to start a session when she very matter-of-factly asked me if I knew what the word "paradox" meant.

"Sure," I told her. "It's like damned if you do and damned if you don't."

Claire felt she was in that sort of situation. She and Vinnie had become close and he wanted her to be his slave. Claire, on the other had, wanted to be with both Vinnie and Kira, something she was certain she couldn't manage.

This upset me terribly, but I tried not to show it. All this time I thought Vinnie wanted *me* to be his slave and he was making the same promises to Claire. Of course, he was also still living with Lila at the time. I was livid, but I somehow managed to go on with my session.

Later, in the back room, I started banging things around and crying. Noel was working as a Mistress at the Chalet. She walked in on me while I was sobbing my heart out. She knew damned well what was going on, but never told me. It turned out that Noel was fooling around with Vinnie too. The bastard really got around! "No man is worth crying over like that," Noel said, trying to calm me down. I appreciated her bit of pity and empathy, but I continued to wail.

Being a dutiful slave, Claire alerted Kevin to my outburst. He came to see what was wrong with me. I told him about Claire and how I wanted to be Vinnie's total slave. "Don't worry about Claire," Kevin said with authority but little sympathy. "She belongs to *us*. No one's going to have her."

At a Friday night party, Vinnie told me, "If you want me to be your Master, I'll be happy to take over. But I have to continue to see Lila. She really needs me, too." I can't believe it now, but I took Vinnie up on his halfhearted offer. As a slave in training, I thought I had to be submissive and show him that I was willing to do anything for him. His terms coincided with the fantasy I had created.

After I proclaimed my devotion, Vinnie and I did a few public scenes together, mostly at Chalet parties. I tried hard to please him, but he paid very little attention to me. After one particularly intense public whipping scene he left immediately to join Lila in another room. Another time he stopped by my apartment very early in the morning on the way to the gym and simply fucked me and left. But everything Vinnie chose to give me was okay. At least it was *something*.

In the meantime, my drinking started escalating. Immersed in alcohol, I was blotting out reality. It didn't really matter. Most of the other girls at the Chalet drifted about in the same foggy state of mind, numbed by one drug or another. Despite my unresolved "relationship" with Vinnie, I was making a lot of money. I had many repeat customers and was successful in that respect, but deep inside I was very unhappy and lonely.

I did have friends. The other girls were very apathetic, and often our waiting times between sessions had the warmth and fun of teenage pajama parties, but in leather. After the night she'd discovered me sobbing over Vinnie, Noel and I became very good friends. She had a similar situation with a guy named Derek, so we commiserated. Noel kept trying to tell Vinnie that he should treat me with more respect and have more regard for my feelings, but he never listened to her. Noel and Derek asked me if I'd be their slave, but I wanted no one except Vinnie. After almost a year of this insanity, Noel took me aside and suggested we tell Vinnie that she was taking me on as her slave until he was ready for me. This way, I'd always have her on my side. I'd have someone to protect me. It was a tempting offer, but I was sure it wouldn't work. The sexual problem was obvious. I still wasn't attracted to women and Noel and I were both self-proclaimed straight girls. But I also knew that a lone submissive at the Chalet had to watch out. Almost like in a prison system, one woman could protect you from all the others. Right now, what I needed most was protection from myself. I began to think about suicide. I really hoped that Vinnie would refuse Noel's offer. Instead, there was more of the usual ambivalence. When I discovered that he didn't care one way or the other, I agreed to be Noel's slave.

Everyone assumed that Mistress Noel and I were lovers. It wasn't true. Our S&M play together wasn't arousing for me; it was more therapeutic and nurturing. She never called me a slut or a whore like

William did. Instead, Noel would tell me that I was beautiful, that I should be proud of myself. Even when she told me positive things it would make me cry, because I felt so unworthy. Every now and again, when a strong adult figure said something positive to me, I couldn't help but burst into tears. Was I reverting to my little girl days and craving acceptance from my mother?

Luckily, Noel gave my life structure when I was feeling vulnerable and was really hitting bottom. I phoned her every day as soon as I woke up. The only time we played together was at the Chalet. I was very good at convincing customers to take us on for double sessions. Noel was very fond of bringing in a bucket of ice cubes and running them all over my body, pretending they were trucks chasing each other around. I'd scream at the coldness and laugh at the childish way this truck play made me feel, as though Noel and I were two sisters playing together in a sandbox. One thing I didn't like was the way Noel was able to whip me heavily in front of others. Even though she was a hardcore Dominant, she reversed roles with Derek in the privacy of their home. The fact that Noel was a secret submissive was something she shared with me. Being a "switch" might ruin her credibility at the Chalet, but I found nothing wrong with indulging in your own desires on your own time. Noel had a softer side, too. A few times I saw her cry and comforted her in my arms.

Vinnie left the Chalet and at first I was sad, but after him there was a procession of hot, new bodies. Charlie was only twenty and extremely cute. He first came to the Chalet as a customer with submissive fantasies but later became a Dominant. I liked being on the night shift with Charlie because he was so much fun but also because he was fun to look at. Then there was Ed, a desk person. He wasn't very serious about the S&M scene or the Chalet itself. The desk people were supposed to monitor the girls, let us know when sessions were over, and make sure we were following the rules. But Ed just wanted to have fun. He loved all of us. He'd be a submissive, a Dominant, anything we wanted, just to please us when we played.

Ed began to come onto me. I was shy because I hadn't been with a man for a few months. Besides that, I was also aware that Noel wanted him for herself. "Don't worry, Jacqueline," she assured me. "There's plenty of him for the both of us." There certainly was. Dark-haired and dark-eyed, Ed had the meaty kind of body I favored—not fat, but definitely something to hold onto. I seemed to be attracted to almost every guy who manned the front desk, perhaps because they were my protectors.

The first night Ed and I slept together we were both drunk and stoned on pot. It was sloppy, steamy, heavy sex, a tangle of arms and legs and mouths seeking each other out all night long. One day Ed was kicked out of his apartment for failing to pay rent and Noel quickly took him in. This was perfect because now he was my slave brother and we could play together at any time. With Noel, he wanted to be more submissive, and she willingly agreed to play top to his bottom. One night, we all went to the movies together—Noel, Ed, Noel's two kids, and me. It felt like family. Noel was very open about her S&M practices with her sons, maybe too open. She'd actually tie Ed up in front of them. Although they were only nine and ten at the time, she felt she had to be honest. Perhaps it was too much for them to bear, because they both ended up in juvenile delinquent homes. My guess is that they were probably ashamed of their mother. She'd walk around the house wearing black leather and fishnet, definitely not your June Cleaver kind of mom. After our very typical movie outing, the kids quickly fell asleep. That signified playtime for the adults. Smoking a joint, I watched Noel undress Ed in her bedroom. She cuffed him, securing his wrists to his ankles. A prime Dominatrix in action, Noel expertly teased him with her body and her words. It was her plan to play Dominant with him, and to have him play Dominant with me— Dominant Dominoes. Guiding Ed on a leash, Noel instructed him on how to fuck me. I would have preferred to be alone with him, but I went along for Noel's benefit. I was embarrassed fucking in front of her, so I faked an orgasm and soon it was over.

On New Year's Eve Noel ordered Ed to take me out while she stayed home and read a book. We proceeded to get shit-faced and have a great time. Although I knew Ed wasn't the man I needed, he was still *something,* something to fill up the emptiness. Sadly, neither of my friends was into spanking me very much. Noel would try to get Ed to do the honors, and he attempted it halfheartedly. It soon became obvious that he wasn't happy with our three-way arrangement. When Noel discovered that he was stealing from her she quickly threw him out of the apartment. "Look," Noel told me, "If you can find a guy you really like, I'll train him. I'll teach him to do the things you want." It was a tempting offer, but not easy to fulfill. I didn't know where to begin to look for my dream Dominant.

10

Addict

There was a bar called "Malone's" right across the street from the Chalet. It was a neighborhood place and didn't attract the best sort of people in the world. I'd often go there to relax before starting a session, sometimes after my shift was through. Sipping a double Kahlua and milk one night, I met Joey, a Jewish guy from New York. Although he was secretive about what he did for a living, he was friendly and seemed to have plenty of money. Maybe he was dealing drugs, but I didn't dare ask. After all, I didn't have the most respectable job on the planet either. Finally, a little drunk, I told him that I worked at the Chalet and that I was looking for a handsome Dominant to share my days with. Joey didn't bat an eyelash. A few nights later we went to a nearby rock and roll club. I was plastered as usual and invited Joey home with me. Almost as soon as I closed the door to my apartment, Joey's hands were molding my body. His tongue found its way into my mouth as he lifted my skirt way up on my thighs. Joey felt wonderful inside me, but after it was over I was sure that I didn't want him to spend the night. I was funny about things like that. It was a personal rule that I usually honored. Early in the morning, I dropped Joey off at an apartment building in Hollywood.

It didn't take me long to realize that I liked Joey a lot. I soon felt really comfortable with him. Our dates fell into a sort of pattern. We'd get high and then fuck our brains out. Joey had Noel's approval and I even had him sit in on a session with us. Nothing seemed to faze my Master-to-be.

Now that I had a special friend to do it with, my drinking and drugging increased again. Joey would wake up in the morning slurping a beer and smoking a joint. He never went to work and I still hadn't figured out how he made a living. But the money flowed. Joey even bought a double membership at a local gym. We enjoyed working out together. Nothing mattered. Joey had money and he had drugs. I didn't care about anything else. He had been married once, but it didn't work out. His wife had left him much the way Daniel had left me. In a drunken stupor once, the both of us started crying. After a short time Joey told me he loved me. In fact, he wanted us to move in together. Maybe it was about time I fled the place where Daniel and I had lived as man and wife—too many memories. Joey helped me exorcise the ghost of Daniel by throwing out some of the junk he'd left behind.

Since Joey was assuming the role of Master, he began making decisions for me. Slowly he took Noel's place. Since I was still having trouble going to sleep, I had begun taking Valium regularly. But Joey insisted that he knew something better—a prescription pill called Ativan. It was very convenient that he knew someone who sold them bootleg. Every day, we'd sleep until three, then get up to work out at the gym. On days off from the Chalet we'd crash until five or six in the afternoon. Most of the world awoke when it was light, but I woke up at dark.

One evening Noel and I had a slight argument at the Chalet. I said something she thought was disrespectful to her. During a show we did that night, Noel ordered me into Slave Position Number One— head up, eyes lowered, back straight. Applying both wrist and ankle cuffs, she put me up on the suspension bar. Noel was skilled at flogging. She could maneuver the whip so that only the tips would brush against my back. Used in that manner the whip would sting but not mark. Although she could get heavy-handed with the crop, she wasn't verbally abusive as many Dominants are. Even angry as she was that night, Noel kept praising me, calling me her "golden slave." She added that one day I would find my true Master and be very happy. Noel's words of kindness made me burst into tears. I thought no one in the audience had noticed, but one man guessed what was happening and was touched by it. He came up to speak with me after the show. A Dominant, he was very interested in getting to know me and pursuing a relationship. This was against Chalet rules. The man traveled in from his home in Colorado many times and even did a few sessions with Noel and me. After each one, it was always the same. He would try to persuade me to be with him, but I was too devoted to Joey.

Alas, Joey turned out to be one of the worst experiences I'd ever had with a man. I was still very naive and never thought about distrusting anyone. I'm sure I've hurt people along the line, but never intentionally, perhaps because I know how bad it feels when people betray you. It may sound simplistic, but I've always felt that people should just be good to each other. It's much easier, so why not? We're all in this sinking boat together. It never ceases to amaze me when someone double-crosses me. Little did I know that Joey was a very polished con artist. I soon discovered that he wasn't actually living in the apartment building I'd dropped him off at that first night. In reality he had been living in a cheap hotel. He had no apartment and no job, but he put up a good front. He had used the last bit of money he had to buy the membership at the gym. Joey played me right. He gambled on the fact that I'd fall for him, and I did. Because of my hurt over past loves, I must have looked very hungry for a kind soul. Not only that, but I was seeking a special brand of man who would control me. What did Joey care if I wanted him to whip me or spank me? He'd hit pay dirt. He'd do anything just to hold onto his meal ticket.

Before I knew it, we were living in an expensive condo he talked me into renting. Joey's aggressive personality and New York attitude appealed to me. He never questioned what I did for a living. Why should he? I was feeding him. Joey was supposed to help me with various duties, like running errands and getting my car tuned up. A year later, the car just blew up, so maybe he pocketed the money and never saw to the repairs. I didn't want to admit the truth about him. Deep down in my heart, I knew I was playing with fire. There was a certain vicarious thrill connected with living on the fringe. I never gave the danger a second thought. Since working at the Chalet was semi-illegal anyway, I gave the okay for Joey to start selling marijuana from our place.

I seem to have the knack of walking away from near tragedies unscathed, like the time the Chalet was busted while I was doing a session. Similar to street gangs, rival S&M parlors would declare war on each other, feuding to secure the best customers. Another club reported the Chalet to the police and we were raided. Undercover cops came in and asked leading questions. Give the wrong answer and you're busted. The police were specifically looking for Nina, Noel, and me. They wanted to ask us for sessions and see if we'd say or do anything illegal. They weren't in session, but I was—naked with a client. Since my friend Matt was at the desk at the time, to protect me, he didn't buzz me to signal that my session was over. It seemed to go on endlessly. Finally my customer and I just walked out of the room, oblivious to the raid. At first, I thought the girls were joking. Sliding down the banister, I was acting crazy and lifting my skirt up like a child. Nina's tearful face told me that we really were being raided.

I discovered later that someone in another club had set the Chalet up, trying to get us busted on prostitution charges. In Los Angeles, as most places, offering sex for money is illegal. Noel and Nina had said something that could be interpreted that way. They were taken down to the police station and booked on prostitution charges. They had to sit in jail overnight. Wearing a tight corset into the cell with her boobs hanging out, Mistress Noel spent the night in the slammer. She didn't break down until the next day, sobbing to me that no one had offered to bail her out. Kevin and Kira didn't care. No one did.

Despite the raid, I continued to do bondage sessions at the Chalet. Nothing riled me. I didn't even worry about Joey. I didn't give a damn if he was dealing drugs, just so long as he was good to me. Every weekend we went on our own trip with a Quaalude or two. I taught him the B&D way and he was a wonderful student. He'd often come to our shows at the Chalet and whip me real hard. Because he'd taken horseback riding lessons as a kid in camp, he knew how to use a riding crop. He wasn't sexually involved in what he was doing, though. The emotional aspect of whipping me meant nothing to him. Deep inside, I'm sure he felt the whole scene was a joke.

Our two-story townhouse was beautiful, probably the nicest place I've ever lived in. It had two bedrooms, two baths, and a drive-in garage. Overlooking two tennis courts, the apartment complex also had a big swimming pool. We were so busy drinking and doing drugs that we never got around to furnishing our apartment. Shortly after we moved in, Joey got a regular job selling stereo equipment. The first month, I paid all the bills, including the rent and the security. The next month was his turn. I assumed Joey had taken care of it until I received a call from the landlord at work. Later, Joey glibly told me, "I must have mailed it to the realtor instead of the landlord." Of course, I believed him. Finally, Joey admitted that he'd lied. He sobbed, staring at me with his big, sorrowful eyes. Like a fool, I forgave him. I was always forgiving Joey for one thing or another. It wasn't long before he lost his sales job. He came home with his face cut up and a swollen eye covered with a patch claiming that he got into a fight with some of his co-workers.

Irv was a dear friend who couldn't stand Joey. However, he'd put up with him just so he could be close to me. During a dry spell, Joey bought some pot from Irv and paid him with a check he'd stolen from me. I forgave Joey for that, too. There was one problem after another. After Joey lost one job he suddenly developed a skin rash and couldn't work. Then he had a bad stomach. Three years before, I had survived a marriage where I'd paid all the bills too, but at least Daniel had never lied to me. I kept hoping Joey would change, but it never happened.

While I was working, Joey stayed home. He liked to cook and he kept the house looking nice. He even unwrapped a lot of the wedding presents that Daniel and I had never used. Joey could make fantastic strawberry daiquiris and homemade spaghetti and meatballs. He cooked good meals and was often good company. Sleeping beside him was comforting, almost like being married. And Joey loved to party with me. Together we'd get blitzed, but, once again, I was just masking myself to reality.

On my birthday, we went to Las Vegas. Joey acted as though he was paying our way. In truth, he'd only made the reservations. He picked me up at the Chalet at four in the morning with some wine and cheese to enjoy on the road. That's one thing about Joey—he always encouraged my drinking. As soon as we arrived he suggested I have another drink. Maybe if I got plastered enough, I wouldn't realize that he was taking advantage of me.

Even though I made it clear that I didn't like the thought of having pets, Joey brought home two kittens. He'd heard me say that if I ever had a pair of kittens the male should be black and the female white. "So the male could be dominant," I joked. And that's just what Joey brought me. Finally, someone was listening to me! Someone cared, or so I thought. Joey named the male "Zaphod," after a character from *A Hitchhiker's Guide to the Universe.* I named mine "Serena," after the porn actress. Within hours I fell in love with my little cats. They gave the apartment a very homey atmosphere. I still have those cats. Although Joey was a creep, the cats almost made up for him.

When the kittens were still young, Joey and I drove up to San Francisco. We were somewhat unconcerned about their needs and often left them alone in the apartment with enough food for four or five days. While we were gone, the shit really hit the fan at the Chalet. Kevin paid us weekly by check. Mine had bounced once or twice over the years, but most of the time I had no problem. Now Kevin was consistently giving us bad checks. A new S&M club called "Club Poses" had opened and they were trying to lure away some of the Chalet's prize workers. This wasn't too difficult considering Kevin's rash of rubber checks. Two Mistresses named Pam and Sylvia were the owners of the new club and a man named George ran it for them. I'd met him a couple of weeks before at a Janus meeting. George spent most of his time ardently trying to recruit me. I kindly begged off, explaining that I was loyal to the Chalet. During my mini-vacation, George lied to Nina and told her that I was going to work for him when I returned. Because of Kevin's bad checks, most of the Chalet staff had left him and started working at the Club Poses. Kevin had lost some of his best ladies: Nina, Noel, and Tantala (whom some people know from porno movies like *Bizarre Encounters* and *Out for Blood*).

I wasn't sure what to do or where to go and wanted Joey to help me make this important decision. He told me to stay on at the Chalet, probably because he wanted to separate me from Noel, fearful she might tell me what a waste of time he really was. In the meantime, Kevin paid me up to date with a good check. Another co-worker named Lisa assured Joey that she'd be happy to look after me just as Noel had. Business at the Chalet picked up after a slight lull. For a while we were very short staffed and I was doing double shifts, making twice the money.

Slowly but surely Kevin hired new girls, but the quality was awful. One woman, named Flora, was a big, fat Dominant with a big, fat ego to match. She had filthy blonde hair, crud under her fingernails, and liked to walk around barefoot. Despite her stomach-turning appearance, Flora's slaves worshiped her and catered to her every need. They loved her and she loved herself, so all was beautiful. Sheba was a street-tough girl with teeth missing in the front. There was an influx of women from the Starlight Dancehall, a club that had just closed its doors downtown. One was Jeri, a terrible woman and a pathological liar. There were a few roses among these thorns, however. Brenda was about my height, and very nice. A French woman named Nannette and I became good friends as well.

Lisa was true to her word and did take me under her wing. I worked many double sessions with her. Unlike Noel, she never hurt me. She just pretended and put on a good show for our clients. That's what life was at the Chalet—a lot of play.

It turned out that many of the Chalet girls who migrated to Club Poses were very unhappy. George was a tyrant. He treated Dolores, his personal slave, terribly. There were times when he thrashed her violently as she hung upside down. It gets me angry when real crazies use the guise of S&M to cover up acts that are plain and simple abuse. Many of the girls who migrated to Club Poses eventually came crawling back to the Chalet. Noel discovered that George was skimming money off of their books and tried to get him arrested. It didn't work, though. The police knew that S&M clubs existed and often dropped in to our establishments. We all knew one of the sheriffs quite well and he was amused at what we were doing. That was another reason I wasn't scared of the law. Back then they seemed to be very accepting of the scene. Like it or not, S&M was a part of life.

When most of the female Dominants left the Chalet, Kevin called upon me to begin doing Dominant sessions. From a light switch (being able to play both submissive and Dominant roles convincingly), I became a heavy switch. Perhaps it was all those months watching Noel, but soon I became adept at tying knots and handling whips and riding crops. It wasn't long before I was doing more dominant sessions than submissive ones.

It wasn't easy at first. Being a submissive was so true to my nature at that time that in the beginning I found the dominance act a lot of work. I wasn't very sure of myself. One Saturday night I was working alone. My orders were to "do" whoever walked in the door. Great! Practically every guy happened to request dominant sessions. One friend, Billy, advised meo, "Just turn it around, Jacqueline. Do to them what you like done to you." It was similar to Cathy's cunnilingus credo. That philosophy worked well except for one customer toward the end of the evening. One of the cardinal rules of dominance is that slaves aren't supposed to look their Masters or Mistresses in the eye. One customer kept staring at me and wouldn't stop when I ordered him to. Confused, I dashed out and conferred with Billy. He laughed, "So, let him look, Sis." I guess even S&M rules are made to be broken. Especially when your "slave" is a lot bigger than you are! Today, I have learned to be a lot more firm with my customers. But if someone breaks a rule, so what?

They're there to have fun and they're paying quite generously for it.

As time went on, the satisfaction I got from game-playing with Joey began to diminish. On my nights off, he acted as though it were his duty to service me sexually. He spanked me or made love to me not because he wanted to, but because he felt he owed it to me. Not only that, but I continually caught him weaving a web of elaborate lies. Perhaps to escape reality, I found myself sleeping later and later. Some Sundays I never even got out of bed. Quite a few Saturday nights when I got home from the Chalet at four or five in the morning I'd stay up and drink alone. When the sun was just coming up, I'd walk by the pool in our apartment complex. Disheveled, muttering to myself, I certainly wasn't a pretty sight. Often I'd exchange harsh words with some of the early risers who were playing tennis as I was staggering home drunk. When Joey finally came home, we'd have something to eat, then get even more wasted on Quaaludes.

One night at a Janus party, Joey and I were pretty sloshed after drinking and gulping down a 'Lude each. Suddenly he started to complain loudly about how Janus members were all stupid and ugly. As I was trying to calm him down, he twisted one of my nipples so hard that no one could believe it. Keep in mind this was a roomful of hardcore S&M people and even they were shocked at his brutality toward me. Suddenly Joey wanted to leave. I learned later that he was kicked out by the head of Janus because he had burst into one of the rooms during someone's private scene. Of course, I followed my man dutifully, trying to explain to him that he couldn't act this way in front of my business associates. That made Joey even more pissed off. "Who's more important, me or them? Where I come from, it's family and friends first. Don't you have a loyalty to me?" He sounded like a Mafia godfather into leather. When we arrived back at our apartment, the argument continued in full swing. Still ranting about loyalty, Joey either slugged me or bashed my head against the wall. (I was so far gone, I can't remember which.) I was terrified and dialed 911. I reached the police but then Joey tore the telephone receiver from my hand and hung up. After a short time, the police arrived—a male and a female cop. They were cold and authoritative. I refused to talk with either of them privately. "Everything's all right," I muttered. "It was a misunderstanding." They soon left.

The next day, Joey went to work. It was Monday, my day off. I was hung over and feeling pretty lousy emotionally. Around seven that night, I managed to get ready to go to Jane Fonda's for my work-out. Just as I was about to leave, the phone rang. It was my friend Irv. He'd been at the Janus party and was concerned about my welfare. At first I was determined to keep my mouth shut. Typically, battered women won't talk about their situations. They just suffer in silence and try to protect their attackers. But Irv kept prodding me, asking me if anything had happened after we left the party. The sincere, concerned tone in his voice made me break down. I told Irv about how Joey had punched me and about the police.

"I want you to pack up your things and get out of there," Irv told me. "Now!"

"I can't do that," I stammered.

"Pack your things and go. Don't you understand? He was violent toward you once. It will happen again. Things like that don't change."

Irv was persuasive, assuring me that his home was always open to me. So was Noel's for that matter. If those alternatives wouldn't do, Irv offered to put me up in a hotel. Anything, just so long as I left Joey.

"I can't," I told him. "Joey owes me six thousand dollars."

There was a dead silence, then a sick laugh. "Let's face it, Jacqueline. He'll never pay you back. The debt will just keep increasing."

I didn't want to believe Irv. I kept thinking that Joey would straighten up. If he loved me, he would. Anyway, how could I just walk out of the house and leave my cats? But when I hung up the phone, I knew Irv was right. I started packing my bags.

It was raining outside. I drove around aimlessly, not knowing where to go and feeling lost. Finally, I stopped at a pay phone and called Noel. Sensing my loneliness, she invited me to her apartment, but when I arrived, it just didn't feel right. She wasn't very talkative and it was very clear that I was disrupting her life.

I wasn't at our place when he came home from work, and Joey probably figured I was at Noel's. He called. As soon as I heard his voice on the telephone, something inside of me melted. I went back to Joey, but I soon discovered that Irv had been right about him. Of course Joey didn't pay me back. The situation just became worse and worse. Every now and again he would chip in toward an expense, but the bills were almost exclusively my responsibility. Between the $950 a month townhouse rental, the enormous electric bills, and the fact that I was supporting Joey's pot habit, all the money I had saved before Joey came into my life began to disappear. My only refuge was drugs. Mostly we just did Quaaludes together, but I learned that before Joey met me he had had a terrible cocaine habit. He claimed that he used to freebase with his wife and a famous sitcom actor. Joey's ex would make him steal stuff from the stereo store where he worked so they could buy coke to freebase every night. Joey asked me if I wanted to try basing. He told me to do it just once so I could experience the unique, euphoric feeling it gave. I couldn't decide whether I liked it or not, but after that first time, I kept pestering Joey to do it again. "You see," he told me, "I bet you never craved another drug that strongly." I had to admit that I hadn't. Welcome to the addictive nature of freebasing.

One day, Joey took my car for a drive. When he returned, he told me a wild story. "Guess what," he said. "The engine of your car just blew up." He handed me a phony-looking piece of paper saying that the car was totaled and that he'd sold it to a junk yard. I never did learn what the truth was, and I never saw my car again. Maybe it exploded because he neglected to give it a tune-up. Then again, he could simply have sold it. We went out and bought a used car—with my money—that night. Boom, boom, boom. That's the way it was. There was never any thought connected with anything. As long as I had some sort of cash on reserve, Joey didn't seem to worry.

On my birthday in May, we planned a fun night on the town. Joey promised he'd play Dominant that evening and really make me his slave. I took the day off from the Chalet so we could have dinner and then go out dancing. I was really looking forward to it. But then Joey came home from work. "I've got good news and bad news," he told me, shrugging. The bad news was that he'd lost his job. Why? Because they discovered that he was stealing. The good news was that he was going to work with his friend Sid, who was in the gray market importing Mercedes cars. He told me that it wasn't particularly legal or illegal, but I didn't understand the logistics of it. Of course, Joey promised me a Mercedes out of his new scheme. But, getting back to the bad news, he couldn't get his paycheck and therefore had no cash to take me out for my birthday. We could still go out if we used the money he'd given me a few days earlier to pay the phone bill. It was difficult enough squeezing money from him to pay the bills, but now he wanted to take it back so we could go out for my birthday.

"Damn you," I yelled at him and then headed toward the door. I'd rather work on my birthday than quarrel with him, I decided. Joey tried to stop me, but I finally got out of his grip. In the car, I pulled over to count the cash I'd managed to grab. Instead of the $250 I knew I'd squirreled away, there was only $50. I knew damned well where the missing $200 was. I started sobbing. Joey was blatantly stealing from me. I finally got a grip on myself and called the Chalet to let them know I was on my way. Joey had just phoned ahead of me. For some reason, I just decided to go home, feeling defeated and numb. I was really angry, but Joey wasn't there. A half hour later he returned with my birthday present—cocaine to freebase.

Cocaine is an amazing drug. I took a hit from the pipe and suddenly felt blissful. All it took was one hit. I no longer cared that Joey had stolen my money to buy the stuff. I even managed to convince myself that he didn't take it. We smoked cocaine all night long. It's a drug that really turns me on sexually. I couldn't get enough dick when we were freebasing, but Joey was usually very busy cooking the coke or fiddling with it. I tried to grab his cock, but he just pulled away. He told me that we'd screw when he was coming down off the drug. It was pretty terrible when the effects of basing wore off. Sometimes sex helped mask the awful feelings inside. Although you don't get agitated the way you do from snorting regular coke, you're not ready to sleep either. Even now that I've been sober for years, I sometimes find myself craving the euphoric feeling that cocaine gives. But it's a very, very dangerous drug and I hope I have the strength never to do it again.

A few weeks later Joey and I had another explosive argument. We had made plans to go away for Memorial Day and Joey had promised to sell enough cocaine to finance the trip. A woman he worked with at the Mercedes place picked him up to do the big coke deal. I suspected that something else had been going on between them, especially when I returned from the Chalet at four a.m. and Joey still wasn't home. There wasn't even a note. I was worried silly. Eventually Joey staggered in and told a bizarre story about getting arrested. This didn't jibe with his admission that he'd been smoking coke all night long, the very same stuff he was supposed to sell to pay for our trip. On top of that, the guy who'd fronted Joey his drug money was actively pursuing him.

No mini-vacation that weekend. I tried to assuage my anger with a Valium and some liquor, but even that didn't numb the pain. I finally realized that I had to get rid of Joey. I was close to having a nervous breakdown. Endlessly aggravated by him, I lost a lot of weight and looked pretty awful. Our lease on the townhouse was up. I told Joey it was time we separated. To my surprise, Joey agreed that we had to break up. He gave me a check for $2,000 to cover expenses. Two weeks later the bank told me that the check was forged. When I pressed Joey on the matter, he admitted that he'd stolen the check from Sid. That was the last straw. Joey could stoop no lower than that in my book. I told him that he had to leave, not at the end of the month as we'd planned, but immediately.

That was on a Friday. I spent the weekend sleeping at the Chalet just so I didn't even have to see him. The room was dirty, windowless, and didn't have any lights, but I didn't care. I would soon be free. I was really looking scrawny and wasted. Some of my clients were concerned and wondered aloud if I was sick. In a way, I was. This was probably the lowest time emotionally in my entire life, even worse than when Daniel left me. Now I was losing my dignity. I let Joey, drugs, and alcohol get me to that point. Determined not to go back to our townhouse until Joey was gone, I was haunted by his phone calls begging me to come home to spend one last night with him. I stupidly agreed. When Joey arrived shortly after I did, he was stumbling drunk. We didn't make love, although we slept in the same bed. I was curled up way off in the corner, dozing restlessly with my money buried beneath the pillow.

I awoke the next morning to find Joey puttering around the kitchen as though nothing had happened.

"You were supposed to move out of here last week," I reminded him.

"I couldn't find a place," he told me.

I offered to give him money to stay in a hotel for a week.

"Are you sure about this?" he asked.

Yes, I was certain. But of what?

For some reason, I felt as though I had to flee, too. I was all set to move out of the townhouse and into a small apartment right near Nina's. I even left a deposit. Lisa came by to help me pack. Looking around us, she asked if I really wanted to leave this beautiful place. After all, I didn't *have* to go. Since I had been managing the rent by myself anyway, Lisa convinced me to relax and stay there another couple of months. Joey had brainwashed me into believing that the landlord hated us, but he was more than understanding when I asked him to change the door locks. After hearing the whole story, he said, "I wish you'd called me earlier. I would have tried to help you." Joey had punched a few holes in the walls. The landlord even repaired them and never charged me. For a few days, I took it easy. My appetite even began to come back. Soon I went back to work. My life took on some semblance of normalcy.

But Joey, damn him, had left me with a cocaine habit. He planted the seed of desire in my body. Before freebasing, I could either take or leave coke. Now I craved it. It made me feel better and although it was illegal, many of my clients blew it during sessions. Lisa was doing a trip with a very wealthy attorney who was noted for having top-quality coke. I was glad when he requested a double session with me. As soon as I walked into the room, he gave me a hit. Immediately I felt euphoric. All my mental anguish disappeared. Not only did I feel good, but I was incredibly sexually aroused. When Lisa came back into the room, I asked her to whip me. My assignment had been to help her whip this paying customer, but I didn't care. She whipped him and me, too. After the session, the customer gave me some extra coke as a present. I took it home and put it away, saving it for a special occasion. What I began to discover was that cocaine helped me do things I was afraid to do when I was sober. It took away the pain associated with Joey and life in general. It helped me function. One night at the Chalet I found myself playing with a guy for free. He wasn't my type and wasn't even someone I'd find remotely attractive when I was straight, but being high made everything look rosy.

Soon, the lawyer's cocaine gift was gone. I made my first purchase from Nannette. Again, I saved it for the right time. Somewhere in the back of my mind I thought I should do a scene with William. Although we hadn't seen each other for a while, we still kept in touch. Perhaps I thought I needed to be whipped very hard to bring out my suppressed feelings. A few years earlier, I remember Mistress Dina being strung up and thrashed by Kevin. At least it succeeded in making her cry, something she couldn't do on her own. I was feeling so numb inside that I couldn't recall the last time I had shed a tear. Maybe that's what I needed.

Knowing full well that I could handle William and the pain of a whipping after a snort, I phoned him. Even though he was a reformed drug addict, he conformed with my desires. "If it will make you lift that pretty butt higher in the air, then you just go right ahead," were his exact words. My little vial of white powder accompanied me to William's shack in the hills. The sensation of being whipped on coke was incredible. It wasn't painful at all, but blissful. William made me look in a mirror across the room so I could watch him whip me. He snapped clothespins onto my nipples, which I normally don't like. Being coked-out, however, I could endure anything. Finally, William gave me a harsh thrashing until I was sobbing. I could cry about everything that had happened to me. Even after William unchained me I wept until I could barely move.

One night I actually overdosed on cocaine. It was a Saturday night at the Chalet, party night. I often tried to party and work at the same time. Even when I was sick, depressed, or had terrible colds, I convinced club owners to let me work. Even through difficult times, the money I've earned has been a sort of savior. Making money keeps me going. That fateful evening at the Chalet wasn't very different. A client came in and asked if I liked to party. You bet—especially if the coke was free and I was making cash while I was snorting it with him. Henry had heaps of cocaine in his pockets. When we began the session, he dropped a pile of powder onto the floor. We didn't even use a straw to do it. Like animals, we were snorting it straight up from the ground.

Henry's "trip" was very easy. He wanted to wear pantyhose while I dressed in a garterbelt, stockings, and heels. He made me lay down on the floor and display my feet to him. Stretching my legs over my head, I caressed my calves and thighs seductively. Then, touching my legs, he'd murmur, "Oh, you're so beautiful. What lovely legs you have." And I'd keep telling Henry how wonderful and sexy he looked in his pantyhose.

"You're such a sexy girl," I'd tell him.

"Do you think I could pass?" he'd ask. "Do you think I'd make money as a transvestite? I could suck a guy off and make money for you."

That scenario went on for the next three hours. We climbed higher and higher as we did more coke. Our rapport seemed incredible. Cocaine gives you the illusion that you're connecting on an ethereal, cosmic plane of thought, when in reality you're drooling incoherently. Billy would buzz us from the front desk, signaling that the session was over. Henry kept extending it hour after hour. He was tipping me $150, which was unheard of. Average tips ranged from $20 to $50 for a sixty minute session. On top of that, I was consuming a mountain of cocaine, which was quickly dwindling. Eager to have some for later, I stuffed coke down my panties and up my stocking legs. In the meantime, I'd leave him every now and then to get us both some water. (Coke users always seem to need ice water.) I was bright-eyed. The other customers remarked about how happy I looked. Toward the end of the session I buzzed Billy and asked him if he could call the Queen Mary and send over one of the transvestites. When Billy asked Kira, she was fuming. "No, damn it," she yelled. "Don't you understand? That's soliciting!"

The next thing I remember was being in the Lipton Room, stretched out on a table. Apparently, I had passed out. Kevin had been trying to rouse me for some time. I wasn't responding to the name "Jacqueline," but finally awoke when they called me Alice. Later I was told that I had walked out of the Queen's Room at the end of the session, fallen to the floor and gone into convulsions. That is a probably the most common symptom of cocaine overdose. The first thing I did when I came to was feel around the spot in my garterbelt for the client's tip. The money was gone. To this day I don't know who took it. After I came to, I was more upset about losing the money than I was about almost dying. Actually, I denied the seriousness of my collapse. I didn't have a cocaine problem. No, not me.

Kira questioned me about what had happened and I had no choice but to tell her the truth. She and Kevin were angry that I'd done drugs there in the Chalet, but I was eventually forgiven. Kira wouldn't let me drive home that night, insisting that I stay at the Chalet. She was probably more concerned that I'd get stopped by the police and that they'd trace me back to the Chalet than she was about my own safety. Next, Kira took away my cocaine and told Sean to flush it down the toilet. Yeah, right! I knew damned well they ended up doing it themselves.

But that bad trip didn't make me stop doing coke. I was very good at denial. No, I hadn't done too much cocaine. It was just tainted coke, I told myself. That's why I had such a dramatic reaction. From now on, I'd get only good coke. In the future, I wouldn't take anything from customers I didn't know very well.

Other frightening drug-related incidents occurred. I had a client named Stan who was a plastic surgeon. He always seemed to have a steady supply of cocaine. When he ran out in the middle of a marathon session he often called his dealer to get more. Stan's trip was transvestism and he had a particular penchant for wearing a garter belt and stockings. At his request, I called him "Sophie." Stan/Sophie enjoyed heavy whippings when he was in drag. I'd string him up and flog him, his white ass exposed in the frilly garter belt. We would play a lot and snort a lot.

"You're not going to tie me up tighter," he'd say. That was my cue to make the ropes even more secure.

Stan/Sophie quickly became one of my favorite clients and I even began to fall for him. Cocaine gave me the illusion of feeling close to the people I snorted with. I played with Stan almost as though he were my boyfriend. But Stan wasn't my boyfriend. He was married. To him I was a pleasant diversion on the side. But to me, Stan was my life. Not only did the coke allow me to let my hair down, but it created lovely fantasy pictures of the way I wanted life to be. One day I heard that Stan died of an overdose. Because he was a doctor, he was also able to get morphine and often indulged in that drug as well. Stan was a nice guy and I felt terrible about his death.

From time to time I'd make drug purchases from Nannette, but the damn stuff was awfully expensive. Alcohol was cheaper and easier to get, especially since it's even sold in supermarkets in L.A. If nothing else, there was always a jug of Almaden wine in my refrigerator. Sometimes I supplemented this with rum. In addition, I was still taking Ativan at night, another wonderful habit Joey had left me with. I had no trouble getting doctors to write me prescriptions so I could get the pills cheaper. At least I didn't have to go to shady places in North Hollywood to buy my drugs on the black market. I was a very organized drug user/alcoholic. I liked to make sure I had everything in advance and my supply was never depleted. That's one thing I didn't like about cocaine. You always had to wait for the dealer to come through, or else go to him to make the purchase. Knowing a drug was within my reach was very reassuring.

I even had the balls to go back to Malone's, the fateful bar where I'd met Joey. Sitting there doing some kind of paperwork and sipping a strawberry daiquiri, my eyes locked with another man's. He was a rock and roll type, a bit taller than me with long brown hair. He was not well put together, almost slovenly, but cute in his unconventional looks. When I got up to leave, he followed me to the door. Erik and I started to talk.

"Do you want to go outside and smoke a joint?" he asked.

"I don't want pot," I made no bones about telling him, "but if you have a toot, I'll take that."

Although Erik didn't have anything on him, he had some crystal methedrine (speed) back at his place. Would I go back to his apartment with him? I decided against it, but we made plans to see each other that Monday night.

It was a drinking date. Right away I told Erik about my fantasies and my work at the Chalet. Alcohol made it easy for me to tell a virtual stranger that I liked to be spanked.

"You mean the way I spank my daughter?" Erik asked.

That was a very sexy image to me. Maybe I like having a "daddy fantasy" because my own father practically ignored me. He certainly wasn't the disciplinarian in the household. Mom was in charge of just about everything, including the thrashings, and, as you recall, there was nothing loving about them.

"Yeah," I told him. "Kind of like what daddies do to their daughters."

Erik smiled and said that it sounded like fun. We wound up at his place and did that little bit of crystal meth he had mentioned the night we met. Since AIDS wasn't too prevalent a fear on the dating scene yet, my big concern was herpes. I'd ask guys quite bluntly if they had herpes or anything else I should know about. Erik gave me a sad look and admitted that he did have the virus. I suppose I looked pretty sad, because he told me, "You seem more upset about it than I am." In truth, I was. I wanted to fuck Erik. Thinking for a moment, I asked if he had a condom. A quick trip to the local drugstore remedied that situation. Our wild fuck was so good that we decided to see each other again that weekend.

The itinerary was totally up to me. Erik gave me the choice of dinner, dancing, and a movie, or a half a gram of coke. You get one guess as to what I chose. Since I had the connection, I picked up the cocaine and Erik reimbursed me. It was a big purchase, an entire gram, one half for us and the other half for me for later. We quickly blew the cocaine, after which we visited an adult bookstore and got porno movies. Erik got so excited watching them that he even started spanking me a little bit.

In those days, it was much easier for me to have a "boyfriend" than it is today. Now that I'm sober, I'm much more withdrawn around men. I'm more selective and I'm not ready to immediately jump into bed with them. I guess because I respect myself more I want others to as well. Today, when I think about whether I could take or leave sex, I decide that I can usually leave it. If I see a pretty guy on the beach and feel attracted to him, my next thought may be, "Forget it." Too much trouble. Too much heartache. Every now and again, I'll let myself go, but not as much as I did in the old days. When I was high, all I wanted was to fuck and fuck. I'd go to bed with just about anybody. It seemed easier to hook up with a guy and stay with him for a while, maybe because I was willing to overlook a lot.

I saw Erik steadily for two or three months, but lately a relationship like that is a lot more difficult to sustain. Guys just don't seem to stick around. Either I easily tire of them or I'm just too busy to deal with the intricacies of a relationship. The majority of the time I prefer my solitude. Erik really seemed to like me at first, though. He had a good friend whose wife, Julie, was an exotic dancer, and he had no trouble comparing my career to hers and accepting it. Because he thought Tom and Julie had a strong relationship, he was confident that we could share a similar one. Erik wanted to get to know me. I was intrigued. You might go so far as to say that I *inflicted* the Master trip upon him. But in little ways, Erik started to become fascinated with the whole S&M scene. If I was a bad girl, he had no objection to bending me over his knee and spanking me. But this was always coupled with cocaine.

Shortly into our relationship, Erik decided to get into the drug-selling business. I fronted him a few hundred dollars to help start him off. He'd deal and later we'd snort up the profits. This is how many small-time drug dealers support their habit. Our relationship followed a basic format. We'd see each other on my nights off, do cocaine, fuck, and play sex games. Sober, I wasn't very attracted to Erik. He wasn't on my level in many ways. During the day he did clerical work at an insurance company. At night he was a rock musician. I don't think he even finished high school, and there I was with my Masters degree. Erik came from a small town in Oregon in comparison to my bustling Bronx beginnings. We had so little in common that it was even difficult to carry on a casual conversation. Whenever I was with Erik, I always made sure to do a little cocaine. Visiting him when I was high made everything seem rosier.

Discipline games were a part of our scenario, and another thing that drew me toward Erik. He was very imaginative and would find different ways, different reasons to spank me. From him, I never received a halfhearted paddling. He'd make up elaborate stories to accompany my punishments. Erik even had what he called a "spanking chair." When he found a dominant role and a scenario that he liked, Erik could easily get consumed by it and go on and on all night.

I found more places to get my cocaine. Nina turned me on to a client of hers who was a recovered cocaine user. Even so, his session included watching girls snort coke. He'd provide the powder and get voyeuristic pleasure watching the women both do the coke and lap each other's cunts. One time he engaged Nina and myself for a session. He licked his lips as we separated the heap of coke into thin lines and sucked it into our nostrils. Then Nina and I proceeded to get it on in front of him, eating each other from head to toe. Another night I snorted alone and he enjoyed watching me masturbate and talk dirty to him.

One major problem with cocaine is that you feel totally euphoric. You lose all sense of reality. When you're high, your emotions are soaring, but when it wears off, you're incredibly irritable. My skin would feel as though it were crawling. I would literally be shaking. There was a sense of being out of control. I felt I couldn't communicate and was on the verge of throwing a temper tantrum.

One night, I did a private session in my apartment with my cocaine voyeur client. Erik came over immediately after the guy left. I had a terrible feeling coming down off that high. Erik cupped my tits in his hands, trying to change my mood. I pushed him away with my elbow.

"I don't feel good," I moaned.

Erik smiled. "I know how to take care of that." He pulled a tiny parcel of coke out of his pocket.

Erik was growing aware of the fact that if he didn't have cocaine, I really didn't want to be with him. I was terribly blatant about it. Erik didn't deserve the way I treated him.

I also continued trying to mold Erik into becoming the Master of my dreams. William agreed to show him the ropes, so to speak. At the time, William had two slaves. Erik and I sat in to observe William in action with one, Louisa. She was really involved in the entire S&M scene and could take an incredibly harsh whipping, after which William would put her in a cage and tell her to masturbate. I've never seen anyone climax with such ferocity. Louisa almost came popping through the lid of the cage. Being whipped and dominated by William obviously turned her on. I suppose she really liked being his dog-bitch.

Erik was an attentive Master-in-training, watching William's every move, asking questions. At one point William strung up both Louisa and me side by side. He pitted the both of us against each other to see which slave could take more of a whipping. The way to play this game was to say, "Yes, Sir . . . may I have another?" after each stroke of the flogger. Finally Louisa quit and I stayed there hanging from the rafters for another two hours. Erik kept asking William what he should do to me. "Just keep whipping her," William told him. By the time we left I was black and blue all over my legs, buttocks, and back. Poor Erik was terribly upset. He couldn't believe I was able to stand so much pain, or that he had inflicted it on me. He was plagued by guilt feelings. As a child, Erik had been abused by his grandfather. The old man ran some kind of preschool in Seattle and was eventually sent to jail for sexually abusing the youngsters. Erik admitted to me that as a child he was not only beaten but also sodomized on a regular basis by his grandfather. Something about our scene at William's brought back those horrible memories.

One night Erik went to my friend Nina's to deliver some coke. They wound up snorting it all together. Nina meekly phoned me and asked me if it was all right if she drove over to Hollywood with Erik to pick up some more. Totally jealous, I shouted at her like a madwoman. "How dare you do something like that? I thought you were my friend!" On and on I went, yelling, making accusations, asking if she planned to fuck Erik. That's how cocaine made me feel—irrational and insane. After I hung up on Nina, Erik called me back and said he couldn't deal with my petty jealousy any more. He kept saying the words "petty jealousy" in a monotone. He abruptly cut off our relationship just like that and began to see Nina regularly. I never knew whether it was just to do drugs or if it had been something sexual.

During the holiday season I was alone again. For some reason Erik changed his mind and told me that he wanted to spend Christmas Eve and Christmas Day with me. Maybe he hated to be alone on the holidays as much as I did. When he phoned, my friend Brenda, her husband Bruce, and I were at my apartment getting drunk. Erik kept phoning, but I ignored him, not even picking up when he spoke to my answering machine.

One day Erik decided he was going to pack up and move back to Seattle. He asked if he could spend one last night together and I agreed. Since we'd last seen each other, I had dyed my hair platinum blonde. I knew Erik didn't like pale blondes, but I didn't give a damn. We met at a bar and kept snorting up in the bathroom. But that wasn't enough for him. Erik wanted to freebase, too. It was 1986 and "rock houses" (better known as "crack houses" later on) were just starting to become popular. Before that time you had to cook the coke up yourself if you wanted freebase. When Erik tried to cook it up, he'd often ruin it. Rock houses made that instant pleasure readily available. It's a good thing I swore off drugs a few months later, because instant crack was too much of a temptation for me.

Back at my apartment, Erik was desperate for more cocaine. "Come on, Jacqueline," he prodded. "You always have a stash." I kept denying it, but Erik knew me too well. Erik promised to replenish it the next day, so I broke down and took out the last of my cocaine. Typically, we began to play our sex games and did coke all night long. Then Erik left. He never gave me back the cocaine he owed me, but he did phone about eight months later from Seattle. After continuous freebasing, he had suffered a sort of mini-breakdown. But he hoped he could quit the stuff and piece his life together again.

Immediately after Erik left town, my biggest worry in life was, "Oh, shit. Where in hell am I going to get cocaine now?" I was used to having it at my fingertips. Now I had to go through Nina and deal with her connection. She was using someone named Ryan. His flower shop was basically a front for his booming cocaine business. The thing I liked about dealing with Ryan was that he'd come to your house with the stuff. It was like catalog shopping for drugs. You never had to leave your own place. The only problem was that Ryan sometimes kept you waiting, a terrible thing for a coke addict. I tried to limit my buying to a gram a week. After a few months it climbed to two grams. I was more obsessed with *having* cocaine at the ready than actually doing it. I needed the control, the power. Not the type of user who had to snort it up immediately, I could save it and ration it out to myself. I prided myself on that speck of self-control. I also liked to carry it on my person when I worked at the Chalet. Just in case I had a submissive session, it helped me deal with the pain.

After a marathon coke session with a transvestite client, I managed to rouse myself for an afternoon Janus party the next day. I could hardly get out of bed. Irv would often ask me out to a friendly dinner, unaware that I was shoveling so much cocaine into my body. I'd often beg off with the "I'm sick" line. This really started to frighten me, because I was beginning to sound exactly like Nina. I didn't want to be a drug abuser like her, but deep down inside, I knew that I was. Although I was ultimately late for the Janus festivities, I managed to get dressed and look fairly sexy in a short leather skirt and a lace top. Although most Janus members were much older than I was, I always entertained the hope that I would eventually meet someone nice there. Sure enough, that afternoon there was one youngish guy named D.H. present. Watching him whip a woman, I told him, "I like the way you work." Very arrogantly, he told me, "Well, then, let me work and come back when I'm finished." His snottiness may have scared another sort of woman away, but it intrigued me. It was almost too good to be true. I discovered that D.H. was a Dominant in real life, a perfect compliment to my submissiveness.

D.H. asked if I was free for the evening. I immediately broke my plans with a French gentleman I'd met at a singles' bar the week before. In the restaurant I took my usual trip to the bathroom to do a few toots. D.H. had recently stopped snorting and was attending regular support-group meetings. Instead of realizing this as a positive attribute, I actually felt badly about it. How I loved to do cocaine and play. Coke was one pleasure that D.H. couldn't join me in enjoying. We made an agreement right then and there. It was very businesslike and nonchalant. I was looking for a Dominant and a lover. D.H. was certain that he could fit the bill. Within moments, this fact was established. We stuck each other into the appropriate cubbyholes. Analyzing it coldly, it seemed as though it would work. At last, it looked like I'd found a Master who appealed to me sexually. Only five foot four, he didn't exactly tower over me, but his frame was incredibly packed. D.H. was a perfectly toned bodybuilder and a curly-haired, gorgeous hunk to boot. His crystal-clear blue eyes made me melt.

Although D.H. was an exception to this rule, for some reason most dominant males don't seem to take very good care of themselves, perhaps because they believe that true slaves should accept them no matter how they look. The norm was for them to be slightly out of shape physically. As a rule, submissive males had the incredible bodies. Of my clients, many are young and muscular with big dicks. I still can't understand why such handsome men have the fantasy of being humiliated, but I am always more than happy to oblige. Two very famous comedians who visited me at the club both enjoyed verbal humiliation.

Maybe it was because they dished it out so much in their acts that they believed they needed to get some back in return. Many times I've discovered that people's trips revolve around the terrible things they do to others in real life. The twist is that they want it done back to them.

D.H. was certainly the cutest Dominant I had ever seen. I watched him finish eating his dinner at the restaurant, not taking a bite myself because the coke took away my desire to eat. We went back to my apartment immediately. Littered with dildos, erotic pictures, and porn magazines, it was a wreck from a session the night before. D.H. didn't say anything about it. We proceeded to the spanking right away and decided to establish a temporary Master/slave arrangement.

The next night, I met D.H. at his apartment. I arrived customarily late. My punishment was to be strung up immediately. My new Master ran his hands up and down my helpless body, scratching me with his rather long nails. It wasn't so much the physical things he did. I got hooked on it emotionally. That made whatever he did seem like much more. For example, at his urging I'd kneel down before him. "I'm your Master and I want the best for you," he'd say as I crouched at his feet. "It's *my* will," he went on to explain, "not your will that matters." That's just the sort of thing an enamored slave wants to hear.

Very early into our relationship D.H. suggested that he manage my money. I didn't like that thought too much. When I voiced my dissatisfaction with that arrangement, D.H. took his hands and wrapped them around my throat, choking me. I started laughing and didn't even beg him to stop. Finally he let go of my neck. "Interesting," D.H. concluded. "You trust me with your life, but not your money." D.H. really liked to frighten me, to push me to see how far he could go. He had a sword collection and he liked to run the sharp blades all over my body. I had no objection. In fact, I enjoyed it.

When the subject of cocaine came up, my new Master instructed me that he didn't want me to snort it unless I told him. Just before his warning, I had just stolen off to the bathroom to do some and his words made me feel a bit guilty. I must have looked awful, like a typical cocaine addict—terribly underweight, listless, and restless. D.H. began to feed me vitamins and protein milkshakes to build me up again. When we went out to restaurants, D.H. would feed me. I liked that, the fact that he cared enough to make me eat. The truth was that I was totally in lust with D.H. and I'd do anything for him. Once again, this was just another elaborate cocaine fantasy that I was creating. Practically the first night we slept together, I told him that I loved him. I'd *never* do that today. And not only did I love D.H., but I really wanted to serve him. In turn, he gave me a chain to wear on my right wrist. It was a temporary symbol of ownership before I earned my collar. Each time I performed an act better, D.H. told me that he'd let out one more link on the bracelet. It symbolized that he would let me go and trust me more and more.

"Welcome to my world and all the challenges in it," read a card that D.H. gave me within the first week of our relationship. He made me keep a slave journal. That's something I had done for William. Private diaries are the only place slaves can say, feel, and vent emotions about their situation. Masters or Mistresses are not supposed to make any judgments on these entries. Most of my thoughts were about the drug and alcohol issue, about how I hoped D.H. could understand that they enabled me to slip into the submissive role more effectively.

I accompanied my Master to a Janus party soon after we began seeing each other. Dressed all in white, I knelt at D.H.'s feet during the entire meeting. We passed around a symbolic crop and the holder had a chance to speak about whatever he or she was feeling while handling the leather. When the crop was passed to me, I explained how happy I was being D.H.'s new slave. I was sure that I'd finally met my ultimate Master and was elated to share my joy with everyone. I felt very proud to be there with D.H.

The first month we spent a few nights together, but our schedules didn't always allow us to connect. One Saturday morning I was fast asleep but dimly aware of the sounds of my Venetian blinds rattling in my second-story apartment. When I opened my eyes, there was D.H. He had actually broken into my apartment! I really thought that he had flown there—my sordid savior of sorts. What a romantic notion.

Fastidious in his habits, D.H. would often get angry if I didn't put a book back in its proper slot on its shelf. If my toothbrush wasn't hung up in its place, he'd simply throw it away. The first thing D.H. did each morning when he awoke was weigh himself. He'd be elated when he gained a pound. Obsessed with losing weight, I wanted to spit when I heard that. But I kept everything inside because I wanted to please my Master.

I did voice my opinions when D.H. informed me that he wanted to become a male stripper. Sure, I loved to fuck those beautiful dancers, but I didn't want my own boyfriend to turn into one. I felt threatened even though I had no right, especially considering what I did for a living. Within a period of six months or so, I had gone from Joey to Erik to D.H. Now I was hopelessly in love with D.H. He was very strict, rigid, and straight. But there I was, loving it, loving him, wanting to be his slave, and wanting to be perfect—and all at the same time. Being perfect for D.H. meant giving up drinking and drugs. It was a thought that really bothered me.

Very soon after, I had no choice but to change my life. It was March 1, 1986, a night I'll never forget. It began like a typical Saturday at the Chalet. I had begun to resent being on call on that particular evening, because it signified a night of enjoyment for most of the population—except me. Stuck working again, I stopped off at a liquor store and picked up a fifth of vodka. I was with Brenda, one of my Chalet co-workers. Although drinking was forbidden on the premises, Brenda and I concealed it by pouring the liquor into coffee mugs and sipping it slow so that it burned on the way down. Sean was at the desk. Since business that night was slow, Brenda and I decided to play with him, especially since we had little crushes on him anyway. At my urging, Sean put a thick rope into my cunt. I showed him how to put it in ever so slowly and then yank it out fast. Vinnie was watching the action and so was Kira, enjoying every minute of our private show.

In between playing with Sean, I was trying to get ready for my Sunday afternoon acting class. I was pacing the floors nervously and practicing my lines. Then, just as I was about to quit for the night, Raphael, a long-standing client, came in. He liked to do a light spanking, and afterward he would hold me in his arms and call me his little girl. It was kind of funny, because he wasn't very old. Hispanic and in his late twenties or early thirties, Raphael liked working girls. There were a lot of clients like him at the Chalet. They'd sit around in the lounge reminiscing about Chalet employees of the past. "Remember what a whipping Heidi could take? . . . Remember how harsh Mistress Papillon could be?"

Raphael decided to do a double session with Brenda and me. I knew it would be an easy time, no need for a few lines of coke to get me through. But, for some reason, perhaps to put on a better show for Raphael, I did some coke anyway. By the time we finished our three-way scene, it was almost five in the morning. Usually I went home alone, but Sean, Brenda, and I decided to go down to the 7-11 for a bite to eat. My car was the first to back out of the Chalet's parking lot. A police car pulled up beside me. I had a very uppity attitude toward cops, feeling that I had nothing to hide from them. I almost began to let down my guard, thinking they'd protect me if anything bad ever happened. Wrong, Jacqueline. Very wrong. One of the officers was very handsome and I had the audacity to wink at him as I backed out onto the street. He looked at me in amazement and called out the window. "Hey, what's your name?"

"Jacqueline," I purred.

"Jacqueline who?"

"Just Jacqueline," I cooed, sounding even sexier.

I was waiting for Sean and Brenda in the middle of the street, my car idling. They dashed over and told me to stop my little game. "You don't talk to cops like that," Sean hissed. Since Brenda was having a problem starting up her car, I gave the two of them a lift to the store. Mildly aware that I had cocaine in my purse, I brushed the thought out of my mind. I felt above the law. I was invincible.

No sooner had I turned the corner than the squad car's red lights began flashing behind us. I couldn't imagine what they were stopping us for and suddenly remembered that I was carrying drugs. They pulled me over and asked for my current registration. I knew I had paid it, but started freaking out. Searching for the papers in the glove compartment, I was losing my composure. The officers could easily see that my reaction was greatly exaggerated, especially in light of the minor infraction they were stopping me for. Actually, the real reason they followed us was that they had seen us coming from the Chalet. Kevin had warned me that one particular cop had a reputation for harassing Chalet girls.

I kept my cocaine in my box of Marlboros. So it would last longer, I usually wrapped it up in two separate little folders. I devised all of these tricks to make a gram go as far as possible. Still searching for my registration, all I could think of was somehow getting rid of the cocaine. I didn't think they saw me reach into my purse and drop the cigarette box onto the floor. But they couldn't help but see that sloppy maneuver. The next thing I knew, all three of us were ordered to get out of the car.

Sean was only eighteen. Brenda was barely twenty. And I'm a big baby no matter how old I am. Literally shaking, we stood on the sidewalk. First, the police searched us. Then they went through the car.

The trunk was full of whips, crops, ankle cuffs, and other assorted B&D equipment. They found a few pills in Sean's pockets and some loose marijuana in Brenda's purse. Last but not least, they discovered my pack of cigarettes under the gas pedal.

I tried not to panic. Stopped twice previously for drunk driving, I was able to charm my way out of it both times. But this was different. Dangling the pack of Marlboros before my eyes, one cop asked, "What's this?"

"I don't know," I said, terrified.

The older cop slipped a piece of folded paper out from between the cigarettes. "Looks like cocaine to me," he grinned nastily.

Brenda was scowling at me. For a moment, I was more afraid of her than I was of the police. She had been a tough street hooker since the age of sixteen and would have happily murdered me for getting her into this. If we wound up in jail, I was sure she'd strangle me in the holding cell. I don't know why, but the police let Brenda and Sean go, but not before they tried to pump information about the Chalet out of Brenda.

I didn't have time to worry about Brenda's wrath. The next thing I knew, I was handcuffed and dragged into the squad car. It was one of the scariest moments of my life, right up there with being raped. My feelings of helplessness were very similar, as though my life had suddenly slipped out of my hands. I was beyond fear. Nothing was in my control. I felt lightheaded and giddy. At the same time, another part of me felt relieved and not responsible for the outcome of the situation.

In a matter of moments I went from being a sexy temptress to being a crazy woman rocking to and fro in the back seat of a cop car. Begging, pleading with them not to arrest me, promising them anything. I was in such a state that I don't even recall being read my rights. I sincerely thought my life was going to come to an end that night. They were going to book me on possession and attempt to sell cocaine. I continued to insist that I didn't know where the drugs had come from.

"I don't know," I kept sobbing. "Maybe it belongs to my boyfriend."

"Just tell us the name of your dealer," the handsome one suggested.

"I don't know anybody," I kept insisting.

The older one kept trying to frighten me even more. "There wouldn't be any cocaine back at your apartment, would there?"

I was so far gone that I suggested there might be. What an insane thing to say! I really did have two grams stashed away there. Maybe a part of me wanted to get caught. I had been seriously thinking of stopping, but didn't know if I had the strength. Even calculations of what I could have done with every hundred dollars that disappeared up my nose didn't give me incentive enough to stop. This horrible experience did, however.

Luckily, the police decided not to take me in for a blood test. That would have given everything away. They did present me with an alternative, though. Either I could sign a warrant letting them into my apartment, or they'd go in anyway, tear the place apart and write a bad report besides. It was a choice without a choice.

I couldn't make my decision. All I could do was cry. In typical good cop/bad cop fashion, the older officer kept yelling at me to shut up and stop crying. The handsome one kept telling me to calm down, swearing that I'd only get a slap on the wrist if I signed the search warrant. I think he was pretty perceptive. He could tell that I had a drug problem and wanted to help me. All the other one was concerned about was getting the lead on a big-time drug dealer. He didn't give a damn about me.

"I'd love to take you to my apartment," I stammered, sniffling. "But I don't have the keys." Actually, this was true because Brenda had both my car and house keys. She was entrusted with my car when I was carted away. But these cops thought of everything. They had the good sense to slip my house keys off the ring before leaving the scene. Their main objective was to close in on all of the cocaine they were sure was being trafficked through the Chalet. This, of course, wasn't true, but they believed it was. They even thought they'd been lucky enough to nab the dealer—me. It was a pretty stupid idea since I was so frantically untogether and unprofessional.

The police pulled up in front of my apartment building. I was numb with fear. At least they were considerate enough not to make a big scene and wake up any of my neighbors. Before we walked through the door, they asked if anyone was inside.

"Only my cats," I told them.

"If we see anything move, we're going to shoot them and then you," the bad cop snarled.

Just like in the movies, the pair of cops burst in through my front door. Sure enough, one of them almost fired a shot—at his own reflection in my wall mirror.

Very obediently, I led them to the two grams stashed in my top dresser drawer. Plus empty wrappers. A pack rat at heart, I had saved every little scrap of paper my purchases were customarily wrapped in. This way, if I ever wanted to calculate how much money I had blown on cocaine, I could do it by counting the bits of paper. With no exaggeration I had almost a drawerful of those damned wrappers. A few days earlier I had contemplated throwing them away, but decided against it. Some of the wrappers still had cocaine residue on them. Evidence. Desperate addicts sometimes lick the papers to get a tingly numbness on their tongues after all the coke is gone. The policemen were diligently writing down everything they saw. There I was, sitting on my own bed, handcuffed and watching them intently. They also found a bag of marijuana. It was ancient, dried out, and not even smokable. They even tagged that discovery onto their report, including the red sifter which was used to grate the rocks of cocaine into powder. My cats were wandering about, looking almost as confused as I felt.

"Do you have anyone to feed them?" the kinder cop asked.

"Won't I be home soon?" I wondered naively.

The bad one barked out a laugh. For some reason, I thought they'd just uncuff me and say, "Thanks," perhaps even tuck me in, kiss me on the forehead, and whisper that it was all a bad dream.

As they led me out of my apartment, I could tell they were disappointed in what they'd found. They had probably been hoping to find a sophisticated drug ring instead of some desperate user's stash. As the squad car whizzed down to the police precinct, I realized that those cops were the first ones to recognize that I had a drug problem. My friends knew that I liked coke, but they didn't know the extent of the obsession it had become. I'd sneak off to bathrooms and snort, so half the time they didn't even see me doing it. I felt ashamed at the way it gripped me. When I wasn't ashamed, I tried to rationalize it. "Nina has a coke problem, not me." Not a week before, I struck up a conversation with a lady named Trudy. A member of Janus, she was also a drug counselor from Australia. I spoke to Trudy about Nina's drug problem, not mine. I didn't have a drug problem. Until I was arrested.

The only people I could think of calling when I was finally booked were Kevin and Kira. After all, they did have a vested interest in springing me because they were worried about whether I'd talk about their cocaine use. Also, I guessed that my employers wouldn't want me detained too long. If I was out of the circuit, I couldn't make them any money. Being dragged into a jail cell had been an awful experience. They had me handcuffed against a wall for hours. It was almost like a B&D session, but there was no buzzer to signify that the time was up. I'd always had prison fantasies, but being behind bars was nothing like I'd imagined it. This was a reality that more closely resembled a nightmare. The police kept asking me if I was losing the circulation in my arms. Didn't they know they were dealing with a pro? "No, no," I smiled like a good submissive.

Finally I was uncuffed and led to another place. "Welcome to your Holiday Inn suite," the matron smirked. The suite was a tiny cell crammed with five other women. I had to go to the bathroom and couldn't wait any longer. It was very humiliating, squatting in front of strangers and peeing into a filthy toilet. One girl was sobbing. The rest of us asked each other what they were in for. Drugs was the common answer. We were all first-time offenders. There was a stark reality about being in jail, not having your shoes. I wasn't sure if my life was coming to an end or just beginning. In my drug rehabilitation program this moment is called "spiritual awakening." Somehow I had a vision of my dead grandmother, the one I had felt so close to as a child. I sensed her presence, that she was watching over me and protecting her frightened baby.

As it turned out, I was only in the jail cell a few hours. Kevin and Kira pulled a few strings and bailed me out. Although D.H. hadn't convinced me to quit drugs, I finally realized in jail that I *had* to stop using cocaine. This was where it had finally taken me. There was no denying that. There was a sense of relief that my self-abuse would soon be over.

I called D.H. as soon as I was released. "If you don't ever want to see me again, I understand," I explained. He didn't say a word after he heard my story. He only said, "I'll come and get you, Jacqueline."

Kevin and Kim sent Billy to bail me out. He had instructions to take me directly to the Chalet, so I had D.H. meet me there. Sitting in the waiting room with Kevin, Kira, Sean, Brenda, and Bobby, I entertained them with my prison adventures. It seemed almost amusing to them in retrospect. They tried to tell me that I didn't have to stop using cocaine, I just had to learn how to use it better. Still terrified, I kept telling them that I wanted to die. I was going to kill myself.

"You can't do that," Kevin warned me. "You're an owned slave.

If your Master doesn't give you permission to commit suicide, you can't do it."

But the truth was that, in a way, I was already dead.

11

D.H.

D.H. picked me up at the Chalet. Over breakfast in a diner, he was amazed when I ordered a champagne and orange juice cocktail. Disheveled and dirty, I hadn't even bothered to freshen up or change my clothes. But I made sure I had alcohol coursing through my body. I made sure of that. Back at my apartment, the lecture began.

"You're a fucking hardcore drug addict," D.H. told me angrily. "Not only are you hooked on cocaine, but you drink booze every day. You can't even shit on your own because all the pills you pop make you constipated. How does that make you feel?"

D.H. didn't give me a chance to answer. He grabbed me by the wrist and dragged me around the entire apartment. Cleaning the place out, he spilled all of my alcohol down the toilet and took away my sleeping pills. He even took my laxatives. Everything. I let D.H. throw away my Ativan even though I knew I couldn't sleep without it. I had another prescription in reserve just in case. Watching D.H., I kept asking myself very seriously whether I really wanted him—or whether I still wanted drugs in my life. It seemed that I had an important decision to make. If I had to weigh all of those chemicals against having a caring man I really did like, I concluded that I really did have a problem. A very big problem.

In the long run, however, D.H. wasn't the right man to help me. He had very little compassion and was very caught up in himself. The day I was bailed out of jail, I went to D.H.'s apartment with him, hoping he'd really want to take care of me. Even though I was still terrified and upset, he told me that he had to leave for a while. A former girlfriend had promised to give him a haircut. Watching TV alone, I wondered if I was worth canceling his appointment. D.H. finally returned and I fell asleep in his arms.

When I awoke the next morning, D.H. took a paddle and started whacking my ass. "This is what I should have done yesterday," he said, swatting me. I'd been waiting for that. It kind of broke the ice, but I was still in trouble with the law. I was booked as a user with an intent to sell the drug. That simply wasn't true. "You've got to go to a drug counselor, or at the very least to a drug program," D.H. said. "You've got to show the judge that you really want to stop doing drugs."

Meanwhile, Kevin and Kira had a lawyer all lined up. They even closed the Chalet the Sunday following my arrest, something they never, ever did. Since I knew Kevin and Kira were angry with me, I felt I had no one to turn to.

The extent of D.H.'s "taking care of me" didn't last very long. I went home the next day, bought another bottle of wine and had a drink or two. Sitting in my apartment alone, I was frightened and needed someone to talk to. With my hand shaking, I dialed the number of the program D.H. recommended. A man named Tim answered the phone. I began to cry immediately. Tim really seemed to understand. He insisted that I come to a meeting that night. Tim was a New York Jewish boy. He had been sober five months and felt good about himself. I could really relate to him since he had a background similar to mine. I decided to go to work late that Monday and meet Tim at the hospital in Culver City, which was hosting the meeting that night.

Driving to meet him, I had a euphoric feeling inside, as though an adventure were about to take place. Tim spotted me right away. A red-haired guy in his fifties wearing glasses, he wasn't the dream man I'd imagined. Although Tim didn't appeal to me physically, he was a very nice person. Because I'd arrived a bit late, he immediately ushered me inside. At first, it reminded me of a Scientology group. Someone named Bob introduced himself to the group. As I listened to Bob tell his story of addiction, I glanced around the audience and was surprised to see a number of familiar faces, people I'd recognized from television, even the lead singer of a popular rock group. This wasn't a bunch of nerdy folks, just people with problems they desperately wanted to overcome.

When the meeting was over, Tim introduced me to some of the women in the group. "You can meet the guys on your own," he smiled. When the ladies heard that it was my first meeting, they were very friendly. They wrote their names and numbers on slips of paper and encouraged me to call them and to keep attending meetings. Everything seemed to progress at a frenetic, sped-up pace, since most of us were hyperactive former cocaine users. Tim walked with me to my car and explained the steps of the program. He said that for now he would be my "guide." I had to call him every day, check in with him to let him know that I was all right, and sober. It almost reminded me of an S&M relationship, of the way I had to phone Noel or William for guidance.

Then I learned something about the program that shocked me. I had to stop using *all* drugs—alcohol, cocaine, pills, and pot.

"You don't understand," I told Tim. "I only have a cocaine problem."

Tim smiled. "You have a lot to learn, Jacqueline. *Everything* is a problem for people like us."

Although the thought of surviving life entirely drug-free wasn't pretty, I decided to give it a try. You're supposed to take it easy during your first thirty days of sobriety. Slow down. Take time off from work. I couldn't. I just couldn't stop working. At the Chalet that night I discovered that Mona had also just begun a drug program that night. Mona's crutch was heroin, but at least we both had someone to talk to, someone who could empathize. Mona would often bring me packages of natural vitamins. One of them actually contained some kind of natural stimulant. Kevin gave us both permission to come in late for our shifts so we could attend our meetings.

I went to sleep that night with a few sips of rum. It wasn't exactly a good start, but at least it wasn't Ativan. The next meeting was at the Cedars. I talked to some people about my sleeping problem and confessed that I couldn't seem to doze off without taking a drink. They informed me that no one ever died from lack of sleep and suggested that I just try it without alcohol. If I didn't sleep, I didn't sleep. No big deal. Since I really wanted to be a part of the program, and also to be around all of the cute guys, I rationalized that giving up drinking was a sort of dues. After all, the program wasn't charging a fee. So I broke my habit of coming home and talking with Nina on the telephone for hours as I guzzled wine. That night I made myself an envelope of Lipton Cup O' Soup and curled up with a trashy novel.

I read and ate until I was tired enough to sleep. I rested better that night than I had in years. I even started to dream again.

I went to a meeting every night. The Chalet continued to let me come in late. During this time Kevin and Kira hired a very heavy coke user to cover the front desk. Brenda and Sean were also snorting lots of cocaine. Apparently their brush with the law didn't make them as frightened as mine had. About two weeks later Sean told me that he wanted to stop doing drugs since they were making him crazier and crazier. It was nice to attend meetings with a friend.

D.H.'s birthday happened to come during my first month of sobriety. I decided to take him to Santa Barbara and enjoy a lovely bed and breakfast suite for the weekend. I felt the same sort of happiness that fictional O felt when she was with her Master—protected, playful, cared for. The only thing lacking in our relationship was the emotional support I needed. Although D.H. had originally suggested that I attend the rehab meetings, he never asked me anything about them. He no longer attended meetings himself because he felt that bodybuilding was enough to keep him strong.

The thought of going to a restaurant and not being able to drink wine frightened me. But it was easier since D.H. was sober, too. He made sure I ordered a full meal and even fed it to me. That weekend was memorable. One of the nights D.H. tied me to the four-poster bed, coated my body with sweet oil, and rubbed his cock against me.

My relationship with D.H. had some semblance of love, but it was far from perfect. Right from the beginning, D.H. was honest, though. He explained that one woman was never enough for him. I could have accepted that, except he was constantly staring at other women even while I was present. If I left briefly to go to the bathroom in a restaurant, he'd already be taking down the waitress's phone number by the time I returned. At the Janus party where I had proclaimed my happiness with D.H, he had met Liz, another potential slave. I tried to put their encounter out of my mind, but soon discovered that he'd been dating her. At the next Janus meeting, D.H. told me that Liz and I would be there together.

"Fine," I said, "but only if I can whip her."

"You're not going to whip Liz," my Master informed me. "You're going to learn to love her."

"I deserve a man all to myself," I told D.H.

This, of course, led to an argument. It seemed we were almost constantly arguing. I found myself getting very ornery. Being sober made me see things all too clearly. I knew one thing—no man was going to treat me like garbage again. But whenever I tried to break up with D.H. I felt so badly about it that I begged him to take me back right in the midst of the attempt.

A week later, D.H. met me after a rehab meeting. He was ashen and had a strange look on his face, so I knew something was wrong. He made me give him back the slave bracelet that had meant so much to me. I suppose I wasn't obedient enough for him. Sadly, I unclasped the gold strand from my wrist. "It doesn't mean we're breaking up," D.H. told me. "It just means that we have to work on our relationship. If I tell you to lie in your bed and stare at the ceiling on your night off, then you do it. Understand?" I knew this was bullshit. Staring at the ceiling wasn't my idea of fun. D.H. and I were on different wavelengths when it came to S&M. His idea of a command might be for me to stop smoking. It was never something sexy. Smoking was my business, not his. My true dominant nature was starting to blossom.

When D.H. and I finally broke up I didn't drown myself in alcohol as I might have done months earlier. I smoked cigarette after cigarette and spoke to Martin on the telephone. He had recently split up with Marlene and we'd become good friends. Although I enjoyed conversations with him, whenever we tried to play, it became disastrous. I kept thinking of D.H. and somehow felt disloyal to him. There was an excitement about D.H. that was indescribable. He *was* my fantasy of handsomeness meshed with dominance. Nonetheless, part of me wasn't comfortable with him. I felt as though I was walking on eggshells whenever I was with him. D.H. was stern, much like a father, but not a kind one.

After D.H., I immersed myself in the drug program. For the past three or four years my only friends had been the women at the Chalet. But most of them were drug addicts and alcoholics, people whom I now had very little in common with. I originally felt very positive in the program, but after a little while my self-esteem plunged. I kept thinking everyone I met there was better than me.

William had been on the program for at least ten years and had warned me not to tell anyone my occupation. But did I listen? No! I never liked living a lie. Besides, I didn't think helping people fulfill their sexual fantasies was such a terrible thing. I enjoyed attending the smaller meetings on Monday nights at Beverly Hills High School. There we all got a chance to talk and it was very intimate. At first I was evasive about my life. I tried to skirt the issue when guys asked why I rushed away after meetings so quickly. They wouldn't have taken too kindly to the fact that I had slaves waiting to be whipped. But soon it became almost like a game. "If we guess, will you tell us?" they wanted to know as we sipped coffee one night. Well, they guessed all kinds of things, from stripper to model to actress. One guy finally said, "A Mistress," and when he did, I couldn't help but burst out laughing. I told them the truth and swore them to secrecy, but of course my coffee-shop companions couldn't wait to spread the word. After that I sensed that people viewed me differently at meetings. They assumed all sorts of things about me and didn't venture to discover whether or not they were true.

About two months later, at a Cedars meeting, I met a woman named Claudia who agreed to guide me in the program. She refused at first, because she didn't think she'd have enough time. But finally Claudia became my guide—and my friend. Something of a social butterfly within the realm of the program, Claudia knew all of the best parties to attend. I needed a drug-free social life, so it seemed perfect, but since Claudia was so popular and pretty, all of the guys flocked around her and ignored me. I was ten years old all over again. A very critical person, she was always telling me how to dress or what color my hair should be.

Sean soon became part of our entourage. We had fun together, but it didn't mask the fact that I was still very lonely. I really needed a boyfriend. The million and one guys I had crushes on in the program all seemed to ignore me. Was it me, or was it my involvement in B&D that everyone seemed to find so unattractive? Very hurt, I even shared these feelings at a meeting.

I suddenly wanted to get out of there, but then someone told me, "Those that matter don't mind and those that mind don't matter." It made sense to me, so I decided to stay in the program. I think part of me was determined not to drop out because of my stubbornness to stay sober. So many ex-addicts become pious and righteous with sobriety. As a result, many hookers give up hooking after they give up drugs. But S&M wasn't like that for me. I didn't become involved in it simply because I needed the money, or worse, money to support a habit. I did it because I liked it. It was a way of life. It was a conscious decision. When I became "better," I would never see B&D as "bad."

Maybe someday the people on the program would realize that and stop trying to pigeonhole me.

Things were changing at the Chalet. Billy wasn't happy that Sean and I were friends. In his twisted mind, Sean stood between him and Kira because he was her son. Billy thought I was somehow trying to worm myself into the relationship as well. To Kira, Billy was nothing more than free labor, but poor Billy had constructed an elaborate, romantic fantasy around his Mistress. For some reason I became Billy's enemy. Soon he was treating me badly, not talking to me or even saying hello. He also wasn't booking me correctly. If one of my regular customers arrived when I wasn't there, he wouldn't ask them to wait for me, but would shove them toward another girl. The Chalet wasn't advertising in papers and they had also begun to look run-down and shabby. And there I was, giving half of my hard-earned pay to them. I knew there were other S&M clubs in the area. Mistress Barbara had her own house and had tried to convince me to move over there. I knew I was a hot commodity. I always made money, so I would have no problem finding work elsewhere. The last straw came when the Chalet got evicted. Kevin had gotten into the habit of not paying our rent, so the landlord wanted us out. Kevin promised the girls that he'd have another place by Monday, a ridiculous pledge he couldn't possibly keep.

It was a difficult time for me. I had just discovered that I was pregnant, the result of a quickie one-nighter. As a result of being sober, I was suddenly fertile. In the meantime, Kevin was withholding our pay. I had to practically beg him for my money so I could have my abortion. That really pissed me off. I gave Kevin a week or so. There was still no money and no new place. While I was waiting, I visited Mistress Barbara's and Lady Jane's establishments. I decided against working for Mistress Barbara because she was a cocaine addict. A lot of the Chalet's regular girls had fled to Jane's—Noel, Tantala, and Nikki. Lady Jane's was situated in a suburban-style house. It was done up all pink and velvety, like a typical bordello. It didn't have the ambiance of the Chalet, but Jane was very nice.

Kevin and Kira were constantly on the phone begging me to come back to the Chalet. I cried and told them that it wasn't easy for me to break away from them. They were very significant to me in so many ways. As weird as it may sound, they were my family, a bad family, to be sure, but I felt a strong tie to them. Just as I knew that I needed to get away from my mother many years before, I knew I had to sever myself from the Chalet to preserve my own sanity. But Jane's was never the same as the Chalet. One reason the girls got along so well at the Chalet was because we were all part of an insane environment. In an insane environment, you have to band together to protect each other from the insanity. In contrast, Jane's had a very "normal," businesslike atmosphere. There weren't many rules or meetings. If sex went on behind closed doors, Jane didn't care. I think Jane was actually amused that I stuck so closely to all the rules I learned at the Chalet.

My income drastically decreased when I moved to Lady Jane's, since most of the customers were expecting extras. There was no sense of allegiance or closeness between the girls. Even Noel and I never became as inseparable as we once were. Perhaps I was growing, changing. I had developed more firm and solid ideas about bondage and discipline that didn't mesh with her beliefs. I never could quite swallow Noel's sanction that she was a hardcore dominant and customers had to do exactly as she commanded. What the hell? It was their money, their fantasy. I no longer believed that there was such a thing as "fixed rules."

Trying to recapture old times, I attempted some double sessions with Noel. One customer wanted to see her spank me, just spank me. Noel carted me off to a room and used a heavy wooden paddle on my behind, literally thrashing the shit out of me. In her warped way, I suppose she was trying to teach me some sort of lesson. She also liked to tell customers that I was a "switch," something I didn't think they needed to know. If they wanted a Dominant, I was a Dominant. If they wanted a submissive, I was a submissive. Customers received their fantasies and I saw no reason why I shouldn't be able to live out mine. The roles I played in my private life weren't anyone's concern but my own.

I felt very lonely at Lady Jane's. It was just a job, there was no doubt about that. I missed the Chalet, but I knew I'd be crazy to go back there. Another S&M club opened in the Valley. The Estate was run by a woman who had learned her craft at Club Poses. The Estate was a place where you had free rein. It was almost as though you were renting out your room there and could do anything you wanted behind closed doors. Noel and I decided to work out of the Estate just one night a week to give it a trial run. It was a logical idea, but basically unheard of in the scene. Each club had a philosophy of loyalty and no girls worked at more than one place at the same time without being labeled a traitor.

Gradually, I began to see that it wouldn't be difficult to build up a customer base of my own. In essence, nobody could promote "Mistress Jacqueline" as well as I could myself. At Jane's we had to pay for our own ads. It was the same policy at the Estate. Despite the fact that it was against house rules, I began publishing my private telephone number in those ads. I wanted to continue to use Jane's place, but I also wanted more control. I wanted to screen potential clients myself. I wanted to arrange my appointments. Reluctantly, Jane agreed. She didn't want to lose one of the most promising Dominants in the business.

Symbolic of the positive changes I was going through, I moved to a bigger apartment. I was hauling around the same stupid furniture I'd had since Daniel had left me, so I decided to start from scratch in the new place, leaving all old phantoms behind me. I met a guy named Howie who built me all kinds of wonderful, functional S&M furniture. Howie started with a bondage table that doubled as a sofa. He went a little wild and added a suspension bar and a sawhorse. At first, my thoughts were that it would be my own private dungeon, a fun place to play with D.H., whom I had begun to see again, against my better judgment. But it wasn't long before I realized that I could start to see clients out of my home and eliminate the middlemen like Jane and the Estate. Since it was a roomy corner apartment with nothing else around it, the cracks of the whips and the sighs of slaves would disturb no one.

A sleazy, mafioso type offered to "set me up," but I realized that I didn't need him. From a frightened slave only a few months earlier, I was becoming a smart, confident Dominatrix and businesswoman. Getting started was as simple as putting ads in the trade papers. My dungeon was already constructed. Most of the sessions were mild (like foot fetishes) and didn't require much extra equipment. Besides, I was beginning to build up an impressive collection of whips, paddles, cock rings, and such. With a $75-an-hour room rental fee for a place like the Estate, working out of a bondage house became a crazy waste of money, especially considering the way things were often run. At the Chalet, they used to rotate the sessions more. The girls would sit in the upstairs lounge and we'd be called down one at a time for a particular client. But at Jane's it was more competitive. Like an old-fashioned bordello, we would sit in the living room and the guys would size us up, shifting their gaze from one woman to the other before they made their decision. Whether you were chosen or not, it was very humiliating. Brenda and I had asked not to be on the same shifts because we feared our friendship would suffer from the competition.

The owner of the Estate didn't care whether I began working out of my apartment, as long as I did occasional sessions at her place. I hired one of my friends as a bodyguard of sorts to sit in my bedroom while I conducted my sessions in the living room/dungeon. He was paid twenty dollars a session just to sit and listen—insurance that no customers would take advantage of me. I worked out of my apartment during the afternoons and did regular shifts at the Estate at night.

I placed ads in the *Hollywood Press* and they turned out to be extremely profitable. My phone began ringing day and night. But nine times out of ten, customers didn't show up. I'd sell my talents over the telephone and give them easy directions to my place. As my client base grew, I couldn't help but feel proud of myself. It proved to me that I could handle all facets of this business myself. On top of that, I was meeting a nicer brand of client, the kind who were more selective, desiring a private Mistress rather than "pot luck" at an S&M parlor. This arrangement worked out well for many months. I was still using Jane's place as my home base. When I occasionally met a customer I had seen at her place, they usually didn't recognize me, since I made sure to wear different wigs and costumes. I also used a different name.

Busy in my chosen career, I quickly found myself getting lonely in my private life. I was going to parties, but I rarely got laid. The submissive men fell to my feet and worshiped me, but there was nothing more, no warm caresses in the middle of the night, no one special to phone when I felt sad. I had a few one-nighters with a string of assorted "rehabilitated" men, but not one of them allowed themselves to get close to me emotionally. I guess they worried that if we got really involved they'd be tagged as weird. True, I had an unconventional career and I enjoyed B&D, but beyond that I was very much like other women. They couldn't seem to understand this. I wasn't Mistress Jacqueline character all the time. More often than not I was simply Jacqueline.

Attitudes haven't changed much, even today. Even when I attend video conventions to sign autographs people don't understand the kind of person I really am. They regard me with a combination of fear, curiosity, and awe, three emotions that don't mesh well with love and understanding. Although I enjoy the very marketable image I've created, another part of me is a regular, old-fashioned person who wants the same things everyone else does.

I don't think of the other me as "Alice," because that's not really who I am either. I still enjoy all facets of the S&M scene, but that's about as far as it goes. I don't want to terrorize a man when I'm alone with him. I don't want to tie him up and beat him, but I do enjoy my work. I enjoy fulfilling my clients' desires. Kinkier people seem more colorful, more open to me. They're much easier to get along with. For some reason, I don't mix well with most nine-to-five folks. Perhaps it's because they're often too busy judging me to see what I really am beneath this thin shield of leather. I'm just a regular woman, that's all.

In my loneliness, I had never stopped thinking about D.H. I finally couldn't help myself and phoned him. He agreed to visit. When I knew he was on his way to my apartment I dropped down on my knees and prayed, saying the "Serenity Prayer" over and over. That's what they taught us in the program. But by the time D.H. arrived, I was anything but serene. When I opened the front door, he grabbed me in the hallway and started kissing me. I unzipped his pants and stroked his cock. Before I knew it D.H. had lifted my skirt. I wrapped my legs around his waist and he fucked me standing up in the living room. Nothing could have been better. There was so much intensity.

But after our incandescent fuck was over, D.H. became his old self again. Even our hot passion couldn't mask what was lacking. He left soon after because he had other plans, but promised to return that night. I was in a constant state of heat and wetness whenever we were together, moaning and staring into his gorgeous eyes as he fucked me. D.H. was the physical personification of my lifetime fantasy. He could have been so much more if only he had been there for me emotionally.

Once we visited a friend, Trudy. D.H. began to get playful with me. Together they stripped me, tied me up, and put ants all over my body. The little creatures were running up and down my legs and scrambling all over my tits in a frenzy. It was awful, but I couldn't help laughing. After D.H. and Trudy brushed them all away, he gave her permission to start whipping me. Ordinarily I wouldn't have liked that, but since it was at D.H.'s command, things were different. Trudy's hands were carrying out my handsome Master's orders. I got on all fours and my naked ass was in the air while Trudy flogged me. All the while my head was buried in D.H.'s lap. I was kissing his cock as Trudy inflicted pain upon me. But I could bear it for D.H. I could show him how much I loved him by taking it all without so much as a whimper. I could also look up into D.H.'s big, beautiful eyes as each lash marked my skin. I could watch the appreciation in his face. It was just like a scene out of the erotic French movie *The Punishment of Anne.* I didn't care what was done to me so long as D.H. was there. I knew exactly where I wanted to be—with him.

After the whipping I knelt down with my eyes closed. Suddenly I felt a wet tongue in my mouth. I thought it was D.H. and returned it with a fiery kiss. To my surprise it was Trudy. I was suddenly unaroused. D.H. started fucking me hard from behind, giving me no chance to orgasm. But somehow it didn't matter.

When I broke up with D.H. the first time, he took up with Liz and Carla, the girlfriend of the head of Janus. During the summer, Liz phoned me. She had a problem and needed someone to talk to. A sweet, cute brunette in her mid-twenties, Liz didn't like D.H.'s aloof attitude either. As he had done with me, D.H. made it very clear to Liz that she wasn't his one and only. In fact, he stressed that Carla was his main squeeze. When Liz became pregnant with D.H.'s child, he didn't even bother to take her to get the abortion. He spent the weekend with Carla. Once Liz had been "the enemy," but now I felt strong compassion toward her. It was almost as though I were her sponsor in the D.H. Victims Club. Talking about him made D.H. even more vibrant in my mind. Although it was crystal clear that D.H. was a bastard, I desired him even more.

I discussed Liz's emotional situation with William. He told me to have Liz call him. It seemed that she was badly in need of guidance and William fancied himself the man to save her—not as a knight in shining armor to the rescue, but as a Master in black leather. Three years later, Liz and William are still together. Although their relationship isn't perfect, it offers a sort of stability so that both get what they need from it. Liz is a lot like me in many ways. A bit younger, she was in dire need of the structure that William gave to her life. D.H. almost destroyed her. If she was looking for a daddy, she certainly found one in William. There are many parallels between our lives. It's as though she followed in my invisible footsteps. When I first met Liz, she had a straight job. Like me, she went from being a "normal" person to being a "working girl." In many ways, ladies who are employed by bondage parlors *are* working girls. It's not my favorite analogy, but we are being paid to perform a specialized sexual service. Even though intercourse isn't involved, the emotional act is very intimate. Like many prostitutes, our spirits often become hardened, and our souls become jaded to life. Like me, Liz enjoys playing in the scene, but William takes it all too seriously for her taste. She isn't into his dog-bitch trip, so they rarely indulge in that role. For one reason or another, their relationship works. Perhaps they genuinely need each other. Something safe and sure, even if mildly unsatisfactory, is often more comfortable than the vast unknown.

Keep in mind that months before, Liz was the same woman I wanted to whip because I thought she was taking D.H. away from me. Talking to her about him made me want to be with him again. I craved his passion. I wanted to be fucked with the intensity that I've only been able to find with a few men. With D.H., everything fell into place. It went beyond spanking. I experienced the ultimate feeling of lust and heat with him, a delicious, wonderful feeling. Knowing it makes me understand why many of my slaves want to be with me, even though they know full well that they can't possess me or become an integral part of my life. At least they can have a small part of me. I'm a catalyst for their feelings. Many of us who desire certain things strongly are often willing to settle for what we can get. A fragment of a dream is better than nothing. Even though S&M isn't always real, the intensity of feeling it gives you makes up for the lack of reality. That's what I was searching for with D.H. I wanted some tiny piece of him, knowing full well that I couldn't possess all of him.

When D.H. and I left Trudy's that night, I felt as though I were in a dream, tripping on the fringes of another world. I was happy to be back with him. A few days later, D.H. visited me at Lady Jane's. D.H. and I had been discussing the possibility of him marking me. That would signify that I really belonged to him. D.H. brought a friend along, plus a scalpel. They were playing with me, poking me. One of my clients was into needle torture, so I had quite a selection at my fingertips. D.H. started scratching me with the sharp points. I was bleeding, but I liked it. I liked anything D.H. gave to me—even pain. Jane was watching our scene in amazement. She couldn't believe the change that came over me when I was with this man.

A few days later, D.H. asked, "How would you feel about calling me 'Master'?" In my heart, I knew that nothing would make me happier, but there was more to it than simply calling him by a different name. When a slave addressed someone as "Master" there were all sorts of trials and tribulations, physical tests of devotion. D.H. wasn't interested in that aspect of the game. He just wanted the power over me.

My response to D.H.'s proposal was, "Yes, Master."

As soon as those words passed my lips, I felt lightheaded, as though a weight had been lifted from me. My committment to D.H. was established and I willingly relinquished the control over my own destiny. D.H. was to make all of my decisions now. He was to lead me. That's what many slaves really crave—to be free of the burden of making their own decisions. A Master or Mistress handles all of those pressures.

"Are you sure that's what you really want?" Claudia asked when I informed her of my pledge.

"I can't do anything about it," I told her. "He's my Master now. It's over."

Wearing chains, I felt totally free once again. I was able to work and be happy just knowing that a part of me belonged to D.H. I loved and adored him. It seemed as though it would be much better this time around, and our arrangement did work for a little while. I knew D.H. had Carla on the side, but it didn't bother me at first.

Shortly thereafter, D.H. went back on the road. We didn't see each other too frequently, but I had something nice to think about when he was gone. Before D.H. left, I did give him permission to mark me. I never actually thought he was going to do it, though. I lay on my belly naked in my bed, motionless, so D.H. could carve his mark on my flesh. I felt a sharp sensation between the small of my back and my right ass cheek. That's where D.H. carved a horizontal question mark. It did hurt, but it wasn't as painful as you might think. Anyway, I was too thrilled, too honored to feel much discomfort. D. H. tended to me and kept blotting my blood until it stopped flowing. Ruled by my fiery passions, I have even kept the tissue stained with the imprint of his mark. True to his personality, D.H. literally rubbed salt into the wound he had made. Then he spanked me, spread my legs, and fucked me hard as a reward for my devotion. I still have D.H.'s mark on my body. I don't regret it, but I do wish it meant what it signifies. In the B&D circuit, when slaves bear their Masters' mark, it is symbolic of their love and devotion. D.H.'s mark turned out to be meaningless.

Shortly thereafter, D.H. wanted me to attend Janus's Halloween party. He made it clear that he would attend with both Carla and me. It would be the first time the three of us would do a scene together. I wasn't pleased with the arrangement, but I had to comply with my Master's wishes. I made sure I looked ravishing that night. Claudia did an impressive job with my makeup. I topped it all off with a sexy, torn dress. When I arrived I felt very confident, and Carla turned out to be kind of straight and plain-looking, dressed up as a nurse. I didn't see them at first, though. The other partygoers showed me a great deal of attention. Out of the corner of my eye I finally spotted Carla and D.H. Suddenly hooked up with my Master, much of the fun mysteriously stopped. I wasn't on my own anymore, but governed by his whims.

The Janus party was held at the Estate, where I often worked. Cages were scattered all about. Perhaps D.H. noticed my dissatisfaction with the situation, because the next thing I knew he locked Carla and me together in one of the cages. "Don't come out until you're friends," was his command. I could really have fun in a situation like that with someone like Liz, but Carla was very cold. At first, she didn't even talk to me.

"So you're really in love with him, huh?" she finally asked.

"Yes," I told her. "Are you?"

"Yes."

We both knew there was nothing we could do about it. I knew that Carla felt superior to me. She was almost gloating, obviously sure that she would get D.H. in the end. She would wait it out like a predatory animal.

Since his present ladies were under lock and key, D.H. began scouting the party for other girls. It was really embarrassing to be locked in a cage, because professionally I was now a Dominant. It wasn't good for my business image! But D.H. didn't care about anything except what D.H. desired. Before he released us, he handcuffed us together. Since Carla was a good deal taller than me, it was tough maneuvering ourselves. D.H. whipped us together and paraded us around the room. I tried to feel something toward Carla, but I couldn't generate the feeling. If D.H. loved her, I rationalized, I should at least try to like her.

Jealousy didn't creep into the picture until he uncuffed us and bent Carla over a sawhorse. Watching him paddle her bare ass, I was furious. Damn it, I wanted him to do that to me! But D.H. was fair, I must

say that for him. After he was done swatting Carla, he did the same
to me. Knowing that I could take a hearty spanking, D.H. whaled
on my behind. Then he put me over his knee and spanked me even
harder with his bare hand. I was squirming with delight and flashed
a glance at Carla, who was regarding our scene with envy.

D.H. took great pride in showing everyone at the Janus party the
mark he'd carved onto my body. Carla looked as though she might
die of jealousy. I bore his mark and she didn't. But today, his mark
means nothing, because Carla is still with D.H., not me. Believe me,
I now know how lucky I actually am.

A few days after the Halloween party, D.H. told me that he was
going to give me something special. Putting me in his car, he blindfolded
me and told me that I was not permitted to speak. He drove for an
hour or more. I had no idea where we were going. Finally the car
pulled to a stop. "I know you don't have to be at work until tomorrow
at six," he said. I nodded, afraid that he was going to leave me in
the middle of nowhere. I still couldn't see a thing, but I heard voices.
British voices. D.H. carried me into a house and put me down on a
sofa. I could sense that the room was very dark. A lady with a lilting
accent offered me a joint, which I declined. Suddenly I was left alone
in the room. Trembling with fear, I was also feeling very excited and
aroused. It was like something out of a bondage novel.

Then I could hear D.H.'s footsteps. Sensing he was beside me, I
grabbed him. "Oh, Master . . . Master," I cried. Angrily, he pulled away
from me. I felt myself being lifted up and then placed down upon a
table. Through the blindfold, I could see the blaze of a strong light.
Then there was a sensation of brief electric shocks against my skin.
The thought crossed my mind that D.H. might be branding me. When
I felt him pushing my legs apart I knew that wasn't what he had in
mind. His cock rubbed against my sensitive cunt. Soon D.H. was fucking
me. I felt the presence of others in the room watching us. I kept moaning and calling D.H. "Master" while he pounded away at me. I loved
the way the word sounded. His cock felt so incredible inside of me.

Then someone removed my blindfold. I looked up, hoping to see
my Master's beautiful face. Instead, I saw that D.H. was slurping another
woman's pussy way above my head. It was Fifi, a woman we'd met
at a Janus party. In the car, D.H. had promised he would give me
a treat. Instead, he was indulging in his own fantasy. I jealously watched
my Master tongue Fifi's pussy. For some reason, he had never licked

my cunt. I wasn't happy seeing him do this to another woman, but what could I do? I simply went with it. The fear of losing him helped me bear the scene. All the while I was wishing D.H. would lavish his attention only on me. It never quite happened that way. I kept hoping to be rescued by a dashing Dominant. It wasn't going to be D.H., I was sure of that. I guess I was beginning to realize the Dominant lived inside me—it *was* me!

Soon after the Halloween party, D.H. went on the road again. Before he left, he slapped my ass gently. "I want you to stop smoking while I'm gone," he said coldly. I was disappointed again. When was he going to start to give me sexy commands—like ordering me to masturbate for him every night, or stick a dildo up my ass as I moaned his name? I told D.H. that I'd smoke as much as I liked anytime I liked. I could see that it intimidated him because it proved I wasn't a mindless submissive. When he returned before the Christmas holidays, D.H. visited me at Jane's, but I knew Carla was living with him. There's no doubt that I was playing second fiddle to her. I was given the dubious honor of picking D.H. up at the airport. But, again, he acted very coldly toward me. He seemed lost in another world.

I was angry. The Christmas holidays were almost upon us. Although I didn't want to be alone again, I knew D.H. wasn't the right person to spend them with. Anyway, he'd probably just stand me up, like he usually did. A glutton for punishment, I made a special dinner for him one night. While he was eating, he stared at me and finally said, "Do you know what, Jacqueline? I truly believe that you're a mental masochist." I was dumbfounded, but D.H. continued with his assessment of me. "It's obvious that I can never give you what you want, but you keep hanging in there." I burst into tears, but D.H. made no move to comfort me.

I made plans for Christmas Day without him. My friend Roger and I planned to go to a party together. As I was getting ready to leave I heard D.H. banging on my front door. I knew it was him. D.H. was the only person who dared to come by unannounced. He knocked relentlessly. I didn't answer the door and just pretended that I wasn't home.

That was it. No dramatic ending. It was simply over.

12

Dominatrix

In March 1987 I celebrated my first anniversary of living without drugs or alcohol. Staying sober meant growing up for me. With chemical dependencies, I reverted to being a weak little girl. Now I was able to take control of my life. My client base flourished. It was easy. I didn't have to split my profits with Jane, the Estate, or the Chalet. As a safety measure, I occasionally worked at Lady Jane's or the Estate, but what I made on my own I kept for myself. One session at my own apartment brought me as much money as two at the Chalet, and I didn't have to sit around all night long, waiting.

In mid-July, the Estate was busted. The police busted one of the Estate girls, claiming that she propositioned a cop who was posing as a client. The next day we all cleaned out the place thoroughly. Sure enough, we found that someone had planted drugs in between the pillows of one of the sofas. The Estate never opened up again. Shanna, the owner, was scared to death. Seeing the Estate get busted frightened me, too. Suddenly, I realized the danger of what I was doing.

By this time, however, I had become a regular in the B&D scene. I attended many parties, "networking," as many businessmen phrase it, showing off my face, my body, and making connections with potential clients. At one of those parties, I met a man named Steve Hawk. He worked for a store called "Singularity," located near Mistress Bernadette's place. She had always been one of my S&M mentors. Even though we'd never met face to face, I knew much about her. Mistress

Bernadette is something of a legend in the L.A. S&M scene. She ran her own fetish clothing store in Orange County and also published a few B&D magazines. Bernadette was living proof that it was possible to have it all. Not only was she a respected Dominatrix, but she boasted a long, happy marriage to a doctor. They even had a few kids. Recently they celebrated their twenty-fifth wedding anniversary with a huge party. Watching them renew their wedding vows was very moving. Bernadette seemed to enjoy her life to the fullest—both S&M *and* the American Dream. Something that I especially liked was that Bernadette invited all of the important people in her life to this special celebration. There were both S&M folks and her husband's business associates there. S&M people weren't censored, but included in the festivities like all the other family members.

Life for me went along very smoothly until May. A few days after my birthday I got into a very bad auto accident. My car was completely demolished, but, luckily, I wasn't hurt. Very shaken up, I didn't show up at Jane's for a week. She never even bothered to call to see how I was.

Since my old bodyguard had been driving during the car accident, I seized the opportunity to take on Steve Hawk as my new assistant. Steve helped me out in other ways. He wanted to interview me for one of Bernadette's magazines. I jumped at the chance, of course. Up until that point I hadn't gotten much public exposure. There was a whole big B&D world out there I wasn't a part of. Steve opened many doors. He did a photo shoot of me for Mistress Bernadette's *Directions* magazine and was very pleased with the results. Since Steve was a submissive, he enjoyed being around me.

I proceeded to walk on eggshells after the Estate was busted. I knew I had to be more careful. Although I usually screened my calls pretty well, one slow evening during the summer I let a client pass through my usual third degree. "We'll talk when I get there," he had told me. When he arrived, everything seemed all right. He seemed a bit nervous, which isn't unusual for a first-timer. When I asked him what he wanted, he was kind of vague. "Reward me when I'm good and punish me when I'm bad," he said. The man agreed to a half-hour session, but then, instead of reaching for his wallet, he went for my throat. I was terrified, and started to scream bloody murder. Thankfully, Steve was in the other room, but as soon as I started to scream, the man ran off and Steve couldn't catch him. When I screamed, oddly enough, the client muttered,

"I knew this would happen." Perhaps he wanted me to overpower him then and there, but he was clearly abusing bondage-session rules—client and Dominatrix *talk about* a scene up front, and *then* we play. Otherwise, it's not consensual. Later, it occurred to me that the guy might have been hoping to start a scene with me. To see if I was a true Dominant, perhaps he was trying to get me to act aggressive with him, kick him in the balls, knock him on the head, or something. I was too terrified to realize it then. Sometimes there's a thin line between a trip and something dangerous. Over the telephone, the man had complained that none of the Dominants he'd encountered were "real." Maybe grabbing me around the neck was his way to test my validity. I was too frightened to see if that's what he really had in mind.

After that experience, Mistress Bernadette had a talk with me. From our mutual friendship with Steve, she and I had become rather close. She was concerned for my safety after the encounter with the wild client. "Look, Jacqueline," she warned, "you're doing something that's very unsafe. You should take a breather and get a regular job for a while." At first I didn't understand what she meant. After all, I had paid for an ad to appear in her magazine and she had promised that I'd get good, reliable clients. But Bernadette suggested I lay low until my ad appeared.

Waiting seemed like forever. I didn't know what to do with myself in the meantime. I actually did start to look for a day job, exploring the possibilities in psychology, but I soon discovered that the job market still wasn't good. Not only were counseling jobs few and far between, but the pay was still lousy. But Bernadette was right. After a brief dry spell, my client base really started to improve.

When I first started, I had no idea how to handle things, but gradually I've been able to build up a business through national B&D magazines. The way I accept clients today is first to encourage them to write to me. That way I get an idea of their personalities, their fantasies. We also speak on the telephone before we actually meet. In the two years I've been on my own, I've kept very busy.

The price for an hour session varies anywhere from two hundred to five hundred dollars, depending on the client and the complexities of his fantasies. For a long time I charged by the session. When I switched to an hourly rate I lost some clients, but as a result I've been able to develop my better clients and stop wasting time with the cheap ones. My clients come from all walks of life, from plastic surgeons to bill collectors. As a rule, they are fairly affluent. How else could they afford the expensive rates required to get one's darkest dreams fulfilled? I try my best to give them their money's worth.

The scene is beautifully set in my private dungeon, complete with candles and soft music. Although many Dominants don't take pride in their appearance, I go out of my way to look alluring. Not only do I keep my body in shape, but my makeup is painstakingly applied. I've often had my hair and face done up for just one client. To me, that's part of the illusion, part of what they're paying for. If a man wants to worship a Goddess, I make damn sure I look like one!

Most of the men I see have similar trips. They want to be slaves. They want to worship a strong, beautiful woman, to serve her, to please her. I play the role of their unobtainable Goddess. I tease them sexually, but am never harsh or cruel. There are many key phrases in the game, the very sound of which arouse slaves—"You're mine," "You belong to me," "I own you." With very few exceptions, slaves are naked during sessions. That represents their subservience, their vulnerability. Perhaps I will give them a treat, bare a breast, or allow them to lap my nipple. But they never see me fully unclothed. Often, they are so aroused at the end of a session that they need to masturbate. Although I don't touch them, I encourage them to relieve themselves. "Entertain your Mistress" is usually the key phrase. Even first-timers know exactly what I mean.

To understand the psyche of a slave, you must realize that their Mistresses are placed on a pedestal. To have sex with them would be to see them, their Dominants, in too vulnerable a light. The dream most slaves harbor is to be granted permission to perform oral sex on their Mistress. To please them with their tongues, to worship their beautiful genitals. For me, this is too private and personal an act to permit. Often, I will offer my breasts or my ass as a reward. They can lap to their heart's content, but my pussy is something I reserve for a select few in my private life. In many respects, it is my temple. It is sacred to me, and therefore not up for sale.

Much like the Dominants I saw at the Chalet, my slaves are a rather bizarre cast of characters. One of my first private slaves was Jason. I'd originally met him at the Chalet. By "private slave," I mean that we don't only do sessions together. I can phone him at any time and ask him to run errands for me. Jason is not an integral part of my life, but he is also much more than just a customer. It took me a year or two to discover that Jason's real trip is hypnosis. He wants a Mistress to play mind control games with him. When we do sessions now, we take turns putting each other into trances. I talk about controlling him. When I say something like, "Do you love your Mistress, Jason?" he automatically becomes aroused. In fact, I've taught him to climax on command, just by hearing my words. I describe beautiful scenes to him when he's in a trancelike state, paint pictures with words about me being in a gorgeous castle served by many attentive slaves. Of course, Jason is one of them. I tell him to think about me every morning when he gets up and every night when he goes to sleep. I tell him to think of me when the traffic light turns red. We have a sort of sexual mantra, a phrase that he says three times before he ejaculates: "I belong to Mistress Jacqueline."

I met Keith at a Janus party. He is one of those clients who prefers seeing a pretty Mistress. Like many of my clients, Keith is married and probably leads what most would consider a "normal" life, that is, when he is not visiting me. For most people, enacting their fantasies through someone like me is a secret facet of their lives. They indulge and then go home to their families. They are very proficient at their chosen careers and at providing for their loved ones.

Keith has a "cigarette fetish." He brings me long, black cigarettes that I slowly and sexily smoke in front of him. When he is with me, Keith becomes my human ashtray. He requests that I flick the soft, gray dust on his skin. Sometimes I touch the burning edge against his cock. Sometimes I tickle it with a sprinkling of ashes. This is all at his urging. I never hurt anyone unless they ask to be hurt. Being my human ashtray is Keith's fantasy and I am paid to oblige. He pays dearly for the privilege.

I see Carl every other month or so. He likes to dress up like a woman. Happy to be of service, I also show him how to apply makeup. Many of my clients are like Carl—closet transvestites. I show them how to dress, walk, curtsy. Sometimes we even dance together or pretend that we're lesbian lovers. Generally these transvestite trips are a great deal of fun. They're like being with a girlfriend. To me, something like a guy wearing women's underwear is such a tame sort of fantasy that I've often wondered why men can't share it with their wives or girlfriends.

Anthony is a customer who lives in Las Vegas. When I was in town for a video convention, I even let him pick me up from the airport. He likes to cross-dress and used to indulge in that fantasy with his wife, but for some reason they stopped the game. I felt a bit uncomfortable when he told her I was coming to town, but she turned out to be a very nice lady. We spoke on the phone and I even gave her advice on how to start up their cross-dressing games again. If more people had understanding spouses I'm sure the world would be a much more relaxed place. People could live out their fantasies without feeling embarrassed, without having to play-act with strangers.

Ernest is a very sweet little old man. Respecting my sobriety, he brings me a bottle of alcohol-free sparkling cider and has a bottle of wine for himself. We sit and talk very amiably for at least a half hour. Ernest usually carries a list of questions to ask me, all sorts of things about bondage and discipline. After I satisfy his curiosity, we go into my dungeon and I whip him. It's a strange combination of being a guest on a talk show and then doing domination.

A number of slaves are into licking feet. Glen, a customer from Dallas, thoroughly enjoys that trip. A bit overweight, he's the only client who refuses to take off his clothes. Besides licking my feet, he likes to rub cream on my feet, legs, and ass. Another client, "Bootlicker Willie," likes to lick the soles of my shoes, the dirtier the better.

There is a particular brand of customer called a "carpet slave." Just as the name implies, they like to be stepped on like human broadloom —but not by a Mistress who is barefoot. The usual preference is to be trodden upon by someone wearing spiked heels so there is some element of pain involved. Perhaps it symbolizes being "stepped on" by society. The difference is that as a carpet slave, there is a conscious choice being made—you give someone permission to take advantage of you.

One very recent and upsetting session was referred to me through a service. Although I often charge $300 to $400 an hour with this service, I have to pay them a $75 commission. All in all, I still earn good money. This particular night I actually earned $900 for a rather bizarre session. I arrived at the house of a man who wanted me to tie him up and then keep feeding him hits of crack from his pipe. Because he was freebasing, his sense of time was very distorted. He kept extending the session and before I knew it I'd earned almost a grand. I saw this client three times before I found out that he was one of the top plastic surgeons in Beverly Hills. Supposedly, one of his masterpieces was one of the stars of "Charlie's Angels." With me he was an incoherent mess, drooling for hits of cocaine from a crack pipe.

Some clients see me a few times a week, almost as though I am a drug they are addicted to. Then, quite suddenly, they may vanish into thin air. That happens quite often in the trade. One client had me videotape him—and that was the last time I saw him! Perhaps seeing concrete evidence of himself on tape sparked some stark sort of reality in his head. It might have hit too close to home actually being an observer of his own session. Clients come and go. I like to think that I give them something they need and that it helps them grow emotionally. Perhaps if they receive it in sufficient doses they are then able to go on with their lives. It's psychotherapy of sorts.

Many people still consider the S&M world unusual, but little do they know that it is quickly becoming the norm. Age-old fairy tales contain aspects of B&D, power play, and cruelty. Think of Hansel being locked up in a cage and Gretel being forced to perform chores. Think of scenes from *The Princess Bride,* or Cinderella's evil stepmother. Didn't Snow White's cruel queen resemble a Dominatrix in both dress and attitutde? What about the martyrdom and suffering made a way of life by many Catholic saints? S&M is all around us, but we don't realize it.

I just finished reading *Exit to Eden* by Anne Rampling. She's a famous author who also goes by the name of Anne Rice. Perhaps most popular for her *Interview with the Vampire,* she uses various pseudonyms for avant-garde works of fiction in the sexual genre. *Exit to Eden* is an unusual tale, a love story in an S&M context. Many of Anne's philosophies are just like mine. In her books she seems to gravitate toward people with alternative lifestyles—transvestites and the like. She professes that as long as people are doing what they believe in and aren't harming others, any type of sexual conduct is acceptable. This way, we unconditionally accept each other without casting judgement.

I really related to Lisa, Anne's main character in *Exit to Eden.* Lisa becomes involved in the S&M scene at first because she is a submissive. She enjoys being overpowered. Even as a young girl she was haunted by dark, sordid, sexual fantasies. But when Lisa finally becomes a professional Dominant, she does it very well. In fact, she creates a multimillion-dollar business. But it all becomes complicated when Lisa falls in love with a very handsome slave named Elliott and takes him away from the sex club. They have a whirlwind romance, but it frightens Lisa. The club owner coerces the both of them to come back. Lisa returns, but feels she's losing her mind. In reality, she is perfectly sane. The strange feeling she's experiencing is merely love. She isn't used to the crazy, confused sensations that come with love and she doesn't know how to handle it.

Anne's novel is very sexually arousing and it stirred a lot of emotion in me. Lisa discovered exactly what is missing in my life today. Real passion! That's the kind of love I need. I'm a wildly sensual, loving woman and I've searched for years for a man who needs a woman like me. D.H. was the last man I could really connect with. Reading about Lisa's quest and discovery of love in Elliott made me realize that there was hope in realizing that perfect, delicate balance between dominance and submission. Even for me.

Lisa concluded that she could have love without S&M and without the role-playing, but I like to think that if Anne really understood S&M, it would naturally enter into Lisa and Elliott's lives again. They could deal with it and enjoy it more fully. Lisa was searching for a man who could love her without having all of those fantasies. Love without all of the extra equipment—whips, crops, and cock rings— getting in the way. That's something I've also searched for, but, unlike Lisa, I want that man *and* the fantasies.

In one scene, Lisa is very confused and the man who originally trained her as a Dominatrix is talking to her. He could have been talking about me.

> You told me that in a very real way, you loved all the sexual adventurers who didn't hurt others, that it was impossible for you to feel any other way toward them. You felt love and pity for the old flasher in the park who opens his coat, the guy on the bus who rubs against the pretty girl, never daring to speak to her. You felt love for the drag queens and the transvestites and transsexuals. You said that you were they and they were you. It had been that way for you ever since you remember . . . It wasn't only that you could act out a scenario of dominance and submission with flawless conviction. It was that you loved. You really loved. Nothing sexual disgusted you or confused you or turned you off. Only real violence, real hurt, the real destruction of another's body and will were your enemies, same as they were mine. You were just what you said you were. But it is entirely conceivable, entirely, that a love like that could not endure forever.

The paragraph struck a chord in me because I feel just that way. Whatever people choose to do is perfectly all right, as long as they don't hurt each other. One of the things that absolutely floors me is that prostitution is still illegal in most states. Prostitution does help certain people and if it were more accepted the health problems it causes could be kept under control. In Los Angeles the police actually look through the sex trade papers and harass the people who place the ads. (That's why I don't advertise locally anymore.) There are gang wars all over the city. Real problems. Why should the authorities bother women working out of their own homes? Sex between two consenting adults shouldn't be a crime. What's the difference if one of them is paying for it? What's the difference between paying a woman $100 or $200 for a fuck, or taking her to a $100 or $200 restaurant, then screwing her after dinner? For some reason, the latter is "socially acceptable" behavior. To my mind, prostitution is a very clean transaction. There's no lying and cheating. Two people have decided what they really want from each other and are honest about it. It's much more truthful than the mind games I see going on between married couples.

Although I don't sell sex, I don't see anything wrong with the venture. I simply don't choose to do it. I know that some people consider me a prostitute. I quickly discover that when I date regular guys. In the beginning, we get along great, but when they find out what I do for a living, it seems that negative feelings arise in them. Just as accountants don't get physically turned on by balancing books, I don't get sexually aroused by being dominant. I like the game. It's an interesting way to make a living, but I honestly enjoy being submissive in the privacy of my own bedroom.

Recently I saw a new client. He's absolutely gorgeous. Although I was very attracted to him sexually, I didn't make him aware of my feelings. It wasn't the time or the place. I didn't want to date him socially because he'd probably want me to be dominant with him and that's not the real me.

I have started writing a question-and-answer column for *Chic* magazine. I like to stress that if you enjoy doing something "kinky," you should be lighthearted about it. You can't start talking about it as though you're confessing a heinous crime. If you approach any fetish in an exciting yet normal way, it makes you feel much better about it. Imagine a guy telling you, "Do you know what really turns me on? Tie me up just a little bit. In a few seconds, you'll see my cock grow really hard." Presented in a positive light, most women would want to give it a try. But when you're ashamed of your fetish, it becomes almost frightening. Filled with anxiety, you might start off by saying, "I know this is really awful but . . . " Who would want to play with you then?

To me, that's what S&M is all about—play. When we're children, playing make believe is all right. In fact, it's encouraged. But when we become responsible adults we have to abandon that. I don't believe S&M is a "lifestyle." That's much too serious a label. B&D is something that should be kept in the bedroom—or the dungeon. An understanding must exist between the participants. A line must be drawn. I don't think anyone should truly control anyone else. If you cross that line in real life, it can become a little sick. There has to be a cutoff point and boundries must be drawn.

Many of the potential clients who correspond with me are very unrealistic in their S&M desires. The truth is that they wouldn't be happy if they ever got exactly what they asked for. I know that's how my own "slave trip" has been. As much as I wanted a special man all these years, somehow I have never found him. One reason is that I picked men who weren't capable of giving me what I wanted. That should have been obvious to me with Vinnie. If he really wanted a slave, he could have had me. Instead, he wasted his time with Lila, a woman who didn't even play slave games, and then it was on to Noel, who made a mockery of the Master/slave trip. D.H. could play the game, but only on his terms. He didn't have the capacity or the sincerity to stick with one woman or develop a relationship.

Today, I'm not so sure I can sustain a "relationship" with anyone. I've evolved into a very independent person. I like my freedom. I like living alone. Sometimes I do feel lonely, but in general my life works fine just the way it is. All too often when a man becomes involved in it things don't go so smoothly. One reason might be because I have very little free time.

There hasn't been a major man in my life for a long time. Sure, I've dated guys here and there. For a month or two, it might be serious, but then it just fades. It's nothing to cry about, though. It's been a long time since I cried over a man. It's been a long time since I've cried in general. I used to be very moody and weepy. When I worked at the Chalet, Kevin used to joke that he could clock my suicidal feelings to about once every other month. I still get suicidal sometimes.

Don't we all? But today it's different. Suicide is a method of escape. I often think about the fact that I really don't want to live too long. I have a few more years until I reach forty, but even that seems too fucking old sometimes. Inside, I still feel like a child. I find myself being attracted to men much younger than myself. Perhaps as an attempt to recapture my lost youth, I often find myself falling for boys in their early twenties.

Recently a friend set me up with a wealthy chiropractor. He picked me up in a big, black Mercedes and we went out for drinks in Beverly Hills. Divorced only a year, he took me to his twenty-two-room mansion. I liked him, but for some reason he never called me again. When I told my parents about this perfect, rich, Jewish doctor, my mother said, "Well, Alice, that's not the kind of man for you." Why not? I wondered. Was it because he was too good for me? I was adequate, but not great. That's exactly the way Randy had appeared to me— adequate, but not great.

One thing that bolsters my emotions is meeting other people in the erotic entertainment industry who share my goals. Through contacting writer, actress, and photographer Annie Sprinkle, I got in touch with Xaviera Hollander. She, in turn, gave me the numbers of some people who might help me get some work in Europe. Years ago I would have never thought that I could be friends with someone of Xaviera's stature. The Happy Hooker herself! Then I found myself working on my memoirs with another of my mentors, Robert Rimmer.

Part of my emotional growth can be credited to going public about S&M. Determined to make it acceptable and to make society understand, I sat down and wrote letters to all sorts of talk show hosts, even Johnny Carson. A few days later, I had a response from "The Sally Jessy Raphael Show." To date I've been a guest twice on that show, once with a slave in tow. I've also appeared on the "Joan Rivers Show." I've also finally realized that not only am I a good person, but I'm also beautiful on the outside. I've tried to transcend the terrible things my mother told me as a child. A man who has really helped with my physical self-image is my makeup artist and hairdresser, Eldon. I met him when I was buying a wig. I knew from the beginning that he was queer as can be . . . the prototype of a gay man swishing about with a limp wrist. But there was also something very amusing about him. I went back to the wig shop a few times, but I didn't see Eldon. Then he called me out of the blue and told me that he was now a hairdresser. The first time I visited him I was amazed at what he could do with me. My very fine, baby-thin hair has traditionally been unworkable, but Eldon can transform me into a wild-tressed vixen.

At first, I thought Eldon was quite flaky and undependable, but I soon discovered that he's very sincere and fun to be with. I joined him and some of his friends in the Gay Pride Parade. Although we had a good time, I quickly learned what a crude bunch drag queens can be. They might greet each other in the calmest of voices, but then utter scathing remarks.

"Miss Thing, look at that guy. He's got such a sorry-looking cock, I wouldn't suck it with a Hoover vacuum cleaner. And his mentality is shorter than a pigeon's dick."

I've noticed that gay men often pick up women's worst attributes, cattiness and jealousy. Recently, Eldon and I parted ways because he's unnaturally jealous of all of the attention I get. In the past, he's flared up on video shoots and even stormed out right before a photo layout, leaving me high and dry and in need of a makeup person. But when he was at his best, Eldon was like a dear girlfriend. In addition to a special brand of camaraderie, he also worked wonders with my looks. "The Sally Jessy Raphael Show" even agreed to fly him out to do my hair and makeup, and so did the "Good Day Show" in Boston. Eldon did my makeup and hair before my first big photo shoot for *Reflections*. I couldn't believe the transformation. I'd seen makeovers in publications like *Cosmopolitan* and *Seventeen* when I was a kid and always believed that I had potential. "You know, girl," Eldon told me quite sincerely, "you could be a *Playboy* centerfold." Where was he when my ego *really* needed him? But he is right about one thing. The way you look on the outside does affect the way you feel on the inside.

I recently discovered a man who did beautiful leather work and hired him to make me custom outfits. They made a remarkable difference in my appearance. Before I met him I had been floundering around, searching for a special look. It wasn't that I didn't spend enough money, just that I was dealing with the wrong people. Form-fitting leather minidresses, jackets studded with stones or little handcuffs, thigh-high boots—things such as these help form a definite image. For Mistress Jacqueline, it's a delicate balance of leather and lace, sternness and softness.

It's important for a Dominatrix to create a "look," because most of this business is public relations. Customers size you up and try to figure out if you're the one to help them live out their fantasies. If you're not, they simply move on. Some go for severe-looking Dominants, while others want pretty ladies. It's all a matter of personal preference.

Women have always been taught to share their men's interests. I remember hearing time and time again that if your husband likes sports, then you should read *Sports Illustrated.* What's the difference between that and helping your man dress up in women's clothing if that's his fetish? Learn a little about that, too. The same goes for men and their women's fantasies. We should all try to understand each other's deep, dark secrets. Maybe, as peaceful residents of the same planet, we'll learn to accept each other and like each other more, instead of passing judgment. We should all dare to be what we really want to be.

I have recently made my business bicoastal. I have a major clientele in New York City. I have created a mail order business that is firm and I hope will grow. Through the mail I offer such items as video tapes, photo sets, worn panties, and a well-defined Postal Slave Training Program. Readers can write me for more information at Suite 350, P.O. Box 4351, Hollywood, California 90078. I also now have two fantasy and fetish phone lines. The 1-900 numbers in California are 303-5552 and 330-5554. The line is also available in New York City (area codes 212, 718, 914, and 515). The number is 970-5552. If all goes well, I plan to have a national 900 number soon offering taped counseling messages. I am hoping to establish myself as an educator and media person for those involved in alternative sexual lifestyles.

I also now have a weekly column in the L.A. *X . . . Press.* I write each month for *Chic* magazine, and I am a regular contributor to *Dominant Mystique* and *Corporal.*

I've done two porno films—*Savage Female Warriors of Burbank* and *Painted.* They were girl-girl scenes, one with Bionca, the other with Sharon Cain, and both received excellent reviews. I'm still a virgin in boy-girl scenes, but if the right part and the right money come along, I'll go for it. I am very well-known in the X-rated industry and have tried to fill in the gap between hardcore and bondage videos. I hope to produce my own S&M videos soon.

Today I don't "play out" my dominance. I *am* a Dominant. I don't "make believe" I am a Goddess. I *am one.* I have grown a lot. It is almost as if the scene took me from childhood to adolescence and finally to adulthood. In fact, that is not only true of me but of the scene in general. You can call that the unpublicized therapeutic aspects of the scene—it really can re-parent and nurture if done correctly.

I now live my life according to my own wishes, needs, and desires. I am truly my own woman. Though I still might crave a few swats on my ass in the heat of passion, that part of me is reserved only for the bedroom under certain rare conditions. I haven't played that way in a long time, though I don't say or even want to say it won't ever happen again. I do know I will never again address any man as "Master"—it simply isn't me and I really don't feel that I am a submissive at all any more. That's a part of my past I have outgrown, just as I did drinking, drugging, and eating to excess. I am now in control of my life and my destiny.

I do have a number of slaves who are pick of the litter. I care for them very much and really appreciate the fact that they love me, adore me, and serve me in any way I wish. I try hard to let them know they are valued, because they are. I don't ever want them to feel emotionally abused the way I did in that position. A few special ones wear my own personal mark—a tattoo shaped like a whip curled around to form the initial "J."

My new fantasy and goal is to help other people as an educator and a visible media person. I am proud to be me. I am public about who I am. I no longer seek approval or disapproval. I have a few good, close friends. I am open to the people I meet. If they like me, fine; if they don't, that's okay, too. My journey into chains and bondage, incredibly, has set me free!

Afterword

Before Cathy Tavel and I completed Jerry Butler's autobiography, *Raw Talent,* I proposed to her that we could convince ten to twelve female porno stars to let us use the same approach. We could put together a unique book—*For Love and Money,* which would explore, in twenty or thirty pages each, how these women, who often come from Catholic or fundamentalist religious families, had managed to abandon their parental sexual and religious conditioning about exposing their bodies and the privacy of sexmaking.

Far beyond prostitution, which is usually a one-to-one private transaction in which the identity of the woman is often not known, porno actresses have to acquire hard-fibered, totally different moral values to get rid of feelings of guilt for transgressing Christian and Jewish sexual mores. How do they survive in the "straight" world of men and women who can't wait to see the sexual teases of women like Madonna or who buy or rent adult films, but have little sympathy for the Eve aspect of women who use their bodies to make money or as a way of life?

Our proposal to female adult film stars was that they would, as Jerry Butler did, talk on tape, and tell about their lives in chronological order. In the process they could answer about fifty questions we felt were in the minds of most men and women who watched adult films.

Hyapatia Lee, Angel Kelly, and Mistress Jacqueline were the only three who responded. Hyapatia, who has American Indian blood, is married to Bud Lee. A beautiful woman, she has two children. Her philosophy of sex and how she manages her marital life while fucking on camera with many other men is fascinating reading. Angel Kelly is the reigning queen of black porn starlets, intelligent, gutsy, and sweet.

But Mistress Jacqueline, whom I had never heard of and who had never appeared in any adult film that I knew of at that time, is a much more persistent lady. She convinced Cathy that she had a story to tell that would go far beyond the twenty to thirty pages that we had proposed in our original plan. She wanted to write her autobiography in much more detail and needed help to do it.

Frankly, I wasn't too eager to proceed. I had read widely in the area of sado-masochism, but the Marquis de Sade and Leopold Masocher and their writings didn't turn me on. Hanging by my wrists and being whipped by a woman with titties bulging out of her ass-revealing leather clothing was not my cup of tea. Like many men, I enjoyed a woman who would occasionally take oral and genital command of my body, but I had no desire to have her tie me to the bedposts or vice versa so that I could sublimate any rape fantasies I might have. For many years I had extolled in my novels the joys of complete sexual merger, tantric sex, and the ecstasy and loss of oneself possible in extended sexual intercourse that assumes total equality, not dominance or submission.

Halfway through Jacqueline's tapes, if Jacqueline had been handy I would have happily spanked her. For the first fifty pages of the manuscript Jacqueline seemed like Herman Wouk's Marjorie Morningstar, a Jewish girl whose tsuris and rebellion from a dominating mother and a passive father would end with her becoming a plump matron who was president of the local chapter of B'nai B'rith.

Helping people write their autobiographies has much in common with acting—good actors become the persons, real or fictitious, that they are portraying. I could do this and totally empathize with a character or person like Jerry Butler. I began to feel that Cathy (who transcribed the tapes and sent them to me for editing) was much more able to become Jacqueline than I was, more able to identify with her masochism, so I told her that perhaps I should drop out and let her finish the book with Jacqueline. We were in the area of Jacqueline's marriage and the inevitable conflict between a man and a woman who each want to be famous or infamous in their own right, not as adoring wife or husband.

At this point, I hadn't met Jacqueline or even talked with her personally. I had seen a couple of still shots of her dressed as a dominatrix in a hoked-up costume. When Cathy told Jacqueline my feelings I suddenly received a tearful phone call from California. Sobbing (she's a good actress), Jacqueline begged me to continue to work with Cathy to write her story. So that I would know her better, she sent me an hour-long videotape, *Seduced into Submission,* that she sold via mail order to her potential clients. If you haven't seen it, and her story fascinates you, I recommend it to you.

I was hooked! Not as a client for a session where I end up naked and moaning to her to please whip me, but by the "what if?" that has always intrigued me when I'm attracted to a particular woman. What if (with an adjustment for age differences) I had married Jacqueline? Watching her in action on this video and another that she did for Bizarre Video in their *Dresden Mistress* series, and now discovering how she had suddenly found outlets for her sexual and masochistic needs, Jacqueline's story was no longer typical. It was frightening, sickening, and sad. If I had married Jacqueline or her equivalent, could I have responded to her need to be spanked? What would have happened if the game playing ended and the other side of her personality surfaced? Would I have been willing to change places and be her slave?

That's why Jacqueline's story is both sad and fascinating. Millions of us marry young. We don't know who we really are. We are in the process of becoming self-actualized in a sex-addicted society that denies its sexual needs with censorship and prefers visual depiction of death and violence on film and on television to seeing a happy man with an erect penis ready to penetrate a loving woman. Being totally honest with another person about one's sexual needs is not easy. Self-disclosure is a tricky business that can evoke horror and condemnation from a friend or marriage partner.

Through her life, thus far, Jacqueline is still in the process of becoming. If the dominatrix side of her prevails, she might never marry again successfully. One day, because servile men probably aren't interested in being whipped by older women, she may return to her profession as a clinical psychologist. The big question is what would happen if she met a man with whom she could "role play" her submissive needs, and at the same time keep her dominatrix personality in control? It's a question that should intrigue many readers, both male and female, because in our interpersonal and sexual interactions most of us play a continual game of dominance and submission. In a much milder way, many men (I can't speak for women) also discover the joy of pain in an unstructured way when a highly excited woman, on the verge of orgasm, clutches his behind, digs her fingernails into him, or bites and scratches him because she can't help herself, and in the process helps her lover escape his own reality for a moment.

Bob Rimmer

Suggested Reading

The authors hope *Whips & Kisses* has both opened your mind and piqued your curiosity. If you seek additional information on the art of S&M, we highly recommend the following works of fiction and nonfiction.

Carter, Angela. *The Sadeian Woman and the Ideology of Pornography*. New York: Pantheon Books, 1978. An intuitive look at the relationship of sexuality and power. Carter sees de Sade's Justine as the prototype of all "good" women. Food for thought.

Cowan, Lyn. *Masochism, A Jungian View.* Dallas, Texas: Spring Publications, 1982. Jacqueline's therapist discovered this gem and recommended it to her. Insightful, very intellectual, and interesting.

De Berg, Jean. *The Image*. New York: Grove Press, 1966. This was adapted for the screen as *The Punishment of Anne,* or *L'Image*. It is an atmospheric and beautiful portrait of an S&M triad.

De Sade. *The Complete de Sade*. New York: Grove Press, 1965. Almost every work by de Sade equates cruelty, pain, and humiliation with sexual pleasure. Of special interest are *Justine* and *Juliette*.

Ellis, Havelock. *The Psychology of Sex*. New York: Harcourt Brace Jovanovich, 1966. Second edition. An indispensable reference book.

Freud, Sigmund. *The Basic Writings of Sigmund Freud*. New York: Modern Library, 1938. Although the father of psychoanalysis believed S&M to be "deviant" behavior, his observations on the topic are worth exploring.

Friday, Nancy. *Men in Love*. New York: Dell, 1980. Friday's fascinating collection of men's sexual fantasies, complete with her analyses of them. It covers fetishes, transvestism, and sadomasochism.

———. *My Secret Garden*. New York: Simon & Schuster, 1973. Similar to *Men in Love* in concept, Friday takes a gander at the sexual daydreams of women, including rape, S&M, domination, and fetishes. Very intriguing reading.

Gosselin, Chris, and Glenn Wilson. *Sexual Variations: Fetishism, Sadomasochism and Transvestism*. New York: Simon & Schuster, 1980. A good overview written in a straightforward, clinical style and drawing upon case histories and detailed questionnaires.

Krafft-Ebing, Richard von. *Psychopathia Sexualis.* New York: Physicians' and Surgeons' Book Company, 1932. More textbook-style observations, but extremely enlightening.

The Pearl. New York: Grove Press, 1968. A difficult-to-find paperback, but this reproduction of an underground Victorian sex journal is extremely arousing. The birching, or flogging, aspects of S&M seemed to captivate people of the era. "Miss Coote's Confession" and "Lady Pokingham" are just a couple of the frilly, verbose B&D sagas included.

Rampling, Anne (a.k.a. Anne Rice). *Exit to Eden.* New York: Arbor House, 1985. A romantic novel set in an S&M context. Very evocative and skillfully written.

Reage, Pauline. *The Story of O.* New York: Grove Press, 1966. One of the most highly regarded works of S&M fiction.

Roquelaure, A. N. (a.k.a. Anne Rice). *The Sleeping Beauty Trilogy: The Claiming of Sleeping Beauty, Beauty's Punishment, Beauty's Release.* New York: E. P. Dutton, 1983. S&M fantasy novels at their finest. They will undoubtedly appeal to dominants, submissives, and "vanilla" folks alike. Dearly loved by Jacqueline.

Sacher-Masoch, Leopold von. *Venus in Furs.* New York: Privately printed for subscribers only (illustrated by Charles Raymond), 1928. Another classic piece. Supposedly, it was from Sacher-Masoch's name that the word "masochism" was coined. Born in Austria and a submissive, he was a writer in late-nineteenth-century Paris. This is a favorite among many of Jacqueline's clients.

Scott, Ph.D., Gini Graham. *Erotic Power: An Exploration of Dominance and Submission.* Secaucus, New Jersey: Citadel Press, 1983. In Jacqueline's estimation this is the best book written on S&M to date, even though the focus is primarily on dominant women and submissive men. It gives an intelligent psychological and social overview of the B&D arena. Topics include definitions, types of dominant/submissive relationships, how to join the scene, organized groups (i.e., the Janus Society), the S&M church, the party circuit, etc. The dynamics of S&M, such as pain, bondage, humiliation, fantasy, toys, and techniques are also discussed. Scott also explores the commercial world of S&M. She spent time at the Chateau in San Francisco and even spent a day as a "mistress in training." Jacqueline often refers to this book to "bone up" on various points she wishes to stress before making television appearances.

Sellers, Terence. *The Correct Sadist.* New York: Grove Press, 1983. Although the narrator, dominatrix Angel Stern, reminisces in this tale, it isn't exactly an autobiography. It's more a half-pornographic creation about the scene. The author refers to herself as the "Superior" and gives an often unreal portrayal of what commercial sessions are like. Rubber, leather, transvestism, golden showers, and other topics are included. As the slave who gave this book to Jacqueline aptly commented, "Some chapters are kind of fun."

Weinberg, Thomas, and G. W. Levi Kamel, eds. *S&M: Studies in Sadomasochism.* Buffalo, New York: Prometheus Books, 1983. An excellent chapbook encompassing all aspects of the subject, including essays by Freud and Paul Gebhard. Psychoanalytical observations are juxtaposed with interviews with professionals and others involved in the B&D universe. Unique and educational in its discussion of gay and lesbian S&M.

Videography

During the past few years Jacqueline has demonstrated her special blend of sweetness, beauty, and strength on videotape.

Amazons from Burbank (Valley Girl Productions). Jacqueline's first bona fide adult video. It includes a girl-girl scene with Bionca.
The Dresden Mistress I, II, & III (Bizarre Video).
Fire & Ice (B&D Pleasures).
Leather Lust Mistress (Bizarre Video).
Painted (In Hand Video).
The Night Temptress (Hustler Video). Jacqueline does not participte in the erotic action.
Seduced into Submission. This self-produced videotape was created solely for the enjoyment of Mistress Jacqueline's private clients and depicts an intense session between the loving dominant and her real-life "Slave Doug." Available only through Mistress Jacqueline. Write to her at Suite 350, Box 4351, Hollywood, CA 90078, for further information.
The Sensual Dominatrix (Corporal Video).
Wake Up Call 1 & 2 (B&D Pleasures).